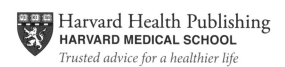

Harvard Health Publishing

HARVARD MEDICAL SCHOOL

Trusted advice for a healthier life

Dear Reader,

Headaches are among the most common ailments that people experience. Nearly everyone has them at least occasionally. Most headaches are minor annoyances. But in some cases, they're severe, chronic, or nearly constant, making them a distressing and occasionally disabling problem. Headaches inflict their misery in a variety of ways, from a dull, steady ache to a blinding, throbbing pain. The most severe types—migraines and cluster headaches—can be particularly vexing.

Even though headaches are common afflictions, they have often stymied physicians. The scientific understanding of headaches was held back for a long time by a lack of a common way of classifying—and therefore identifying and treating—the many types and subtypes of headaches. There's a lot that doctors still don't know about why headaches occur and why certain people are susceptible. But the development of a classification system has been a tremendous help.

Today, we have strategies to help relieve and even prevent many types of headaches. For some of them, over-the-counter pain relievers are effective, especially when combined with rest, relaxation, and a bite to eat. If this approach doesn't help, a number of prescription medications are available, and a handful of drug companies are introducing new medications and novel delivery systems.

This report offers in-depth information on the most common kinds of headaches and the treatment strategies that work best for each, including a number of self-help and alternative techniques, such as acupuncture, which has garnered credibility as a way to help ward off recurring headaches.

This report also explores a variety of preventive strategies, such as using stress management, physical therapy, or exercise in tandem with medications. Another aspect of prevention is learning to recognize and change things that may trigger your headaches—for example, reducing emotional stress, changing your diet, or getting more sleep. It's also becoming increasingly evident that chronic migraines occur in tandem with other ailments—such as anxiety, insomnia and other sleep disorders, or muscular problems. These problems should also be addressed in order for prevention strategies to succeed.

Advances in headache treatment mean that relief is no longer just possible, but probable. Although some form of head pain will occasionally visit most people, no one should have to live and suffer with frequent headache pain.

Sincerely,

Paul Rizzoli, M.D.
Medical Editor

Headache basics

If you suffer from frequent or debilitating headaches, you may have noticed certain patterns. Perhaps your headaches are associated with a lack of sleep, falling barometric pressure, a stuffy nose, or exposure to cigarette smoke. Yet these factors don't fully explain why or even how most headaches occur. Although the pain may feel as if it's in your brain, the brain and skull are not sensitive to pain. Instead, the discomfort comes from pain-sensitive structures—such as muscles, blood vessels, and nerves—in the head and neck. But the precise mechanism underlying a given headache is not necessarily clear. Moreover, it's not clear what function this pain serves. Pain elsewhere in the body usually signals a problem—such as a heart attack, wound, or infection—that needs your attention. But with headaches, in most cases there is no apparent problem to blame—no injury, damage, or disease. There is simply pain.

It was only in recent decades that doctors even developed a common language for describing the many varieties of headaches that people experience. In 1988, the International Headache Society developed the first specific, quantifiable criteria—such as the number of minutes a headache lasts or the number of days it takes to recur—to replace vague descriptive terms like "short" or "frequently." This system, known as the International Classification of Headache Disorders, has been extremely helpful. Before this, it wasn't clear whether one person's "severe, throbbing headache" was the same as another person's "severe, throbbing headache"—and therefore, it wasn't clear how to diagnose and treat it. The hope is that, as science learns more about the causes of headaches, these categories will be further refined, and doctors will increasingly rely on objective tests rather than subjective descriptions to zero in on a diagnosis.

Although mysteries remain, doctors do know a great deal today about the varying symptoms that

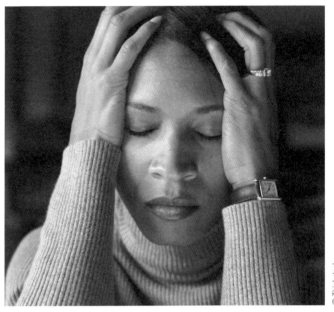

Tension headaches cause mild to moderate pain that is steady rather than throbbing and generally lasts for several hours. Most people feel the pain across the forehead or in the back of the head.

accompany different types of headaches and the triggers that can set them off. Equally important, there are now effective medications to reduce the pain and self-help techniques to help you cope. This report will explain ways to treat headache pain, as well as ways to help prevent future episodes. There are more treatment possibilities now than ever before.

What type of headache do you have?

Physicians distinguish between primary headaches—in which the headache pain itself is the main affliction—and secondary headaches, which are caused by another underlying medical problem, such as an injury, infection, or disease. About 95% of headaches are primary headaches and are triggered by common conditions, such as stress, fatigue, lack of sleep, hunger, changes in estrogen levels, weather changes, or caffeine withdrawal. While headache pain can be temporarily disabling and even frightening, it can be reassuring to know that it usually does not signal damage or disease.

The three most common types of headaches are tension, sinus, and migraine headaches, but there are others. Following is a quick summary of the five main types covered in this Special Health Report. (For others, see "Secondary headaches," page 4, and "Unusual headaches," below.)

Tension headaches cause mild to moderate pain that is steady rather than throbbing and generally lasts for several hours. You may feel the pain throughout your head, but people commonly feel it across the forehead or in the back of the head. These headaches most often affect adults, though children can sometimes get them, too.

Sinus headaches produce mild to moderate pain that is also steady, but which occurs in the sinuses—typically behind the eyes, at the bridge of the nose, or in the cheeks. You are most likely to have a sinus headache if you also have a cold or an active allergy or infection that's causing nasal congestion and discharge. Sinus headaches affect people of all ages.

Migraines produce throbbing pain that is moderate to severe. They often cause nausea and can make you feel very sensitive to light and sound, so that you just want to lie in a dark and quiet room. Rather than spreading across the head, the pain is often localized in one spot—in the temple, eye, or back of the head, and frequently on just one side. In some people, visual disturbances precede the pain.

Chronic headaches occur more than 15 days a month and can be either chronic tension headaches or chronic migraines. Of the two types, chronic migraines are more severe, and they account for more visits to the doctor. They are usually accompanied by other health problems, such as insomnia or fibromyalgia, that must also be addressed during treatment.

Cluster headaches are rare but very painful. They often start in the middle of the night during sleep and

Unusual headaches

In addition to the most common headache types, there are many others, including these.

- **Weekend headaches** are often caused by caffeine withdrawal, which leads to the dilation of blood vessels. This type of headache often begins 12 to 24 hours after your last sip of coffee and is apt to develop on weekends, when you delay your first cup of the day or skip coffee entirely. You can easily identify this type of headache by comparing your weekend caffeine intake with your weekday consumption.

- **Ice-pick headaches** take their vivid name from their identifying characteristic: sudden, brief, and severe stabs of pain to the head. Ice-pick headaches are so fleeting that they're over long before any medication could take effect. This type of headache generally afflicts people who already suffer from migraine or cluster headaches.

- **Thunderclap headaches** strike like a blow to the head, causing sudden, intense pain that peaks within 60 seconds. The pain may begin to subside within an hour, or it can last up to 10 days. These uncommon headaches may appear for no obvious physical reason. But some are a warning of a possibly life-threatening condition, such as a subarachnoid hemorrhage (bleeding around the brain). Because of this risk, you should seek emergency treatment if you experience symptoms of a thunderclap headache.

- **Benign orgasmic headaches** tend to occur in people with migraines and cause a severe headache each time the person has a sexual orgasm. Because the experience may be virtually identical to a thunderclap headache, which can signal bleeding inside the head, testing may be needed to confirm the diagnosis.

- **Paroxysmal hemicrania** is similar to cluster headaches (see above and page 37), but paroxysmal hemicrania attacks are shorter (lasting 10 to 30 minutes) and more frequent (five to 15 times a day). The condition is much more common in women. Scientists believe that paroxysmal hemicrania and cluster headaches are distinct entities, despite their similarity, because they respond differently to medications. Paroxysmal hemicrania may respond swiftly and dramatically to indomethacin (Indocin), a prescription painkiller. The required dose varies, but indomethacin doesn't lose effectiveness over time. On the other hand, it offers little relief for cluster headaches.

- **New daily persistent headache** is a type of primary headache. It is "new" because it develops in a person who has not had problems with headaches before. The onset is sudden enough that a person with this type of headache often remembers exactly when it began. It is "daily" and "persistent" because it then lingers indefinitely. It can mimic either a migraine or a tension headache in the characteristics of the pain.

produce sharp stabbing pains behind just one eye. The pain can be excruciating, leading sufferers to pace the floor, and the headaches tend to recur at the same time—most commonly between midnight and 2 a.m. Most people have so-called episodic cluster headaches that strike a few times a day for several weeks and then disappear during remissions that can last from a few weeks to a few years.

Secondary headaches

Secondary headaches are less common than primary headaches, but they are also more varied. They can have hundreds of different causes. Medications are among the most common. Ironically, headaches can be caused by overuse of painkillers (see "Medication overuse headaches," page 33).

Headaches can also be symptoms of another health problem. For example, a headache may be the only noticeable symptom of a rapid rise in blood pressure. That's why it's important to rule out any underlying cause of a headache that requires treatment in itself. Sometimes the cause is a minor problem, such as a cold that leads to a sinus headache. But in other cases, the cause is serious, such as stroke, meningitis, infection, or a tumor.

When to see your doctor

About 50% of people experience headaches at least once a month, 15% at least once a week, and 5% every day or nearly every day. But only a small fraction of these people ever seek a doctor's attention, since most headaches are relatively mild and disappear on their own or with the help of an over-the-counter pain reliever, rest, or a good night's sleep. But what about headaches that are severe, occur often, or are unresponsive to nonprescription pain relievers?

Although headaches are rarely harbingers of more ominous disease, it makes sense to see your doctor if you're having headaches frequently, if your headaches interfere with your ability to function, or if you have an existing headache pattern that changes in any particular way. The peace of mind justifies the time and expense of a medical evaluation.

Because the following symptoms could indicate a serious health problem, seek medical care promptly if you experience any of these:
- a sudden headache that feels like a blow to the head (with or without a stiff neck)
- a headache with fever
- a headache with convulsions
- a persistent headache following a blow to the head

Table 1: Warning signs that require medical evaluation	
SITUATION	WHAT IT MIGHT MEAN
A headache that's accompanied by fever and a stiff neck	Meningitis, an inflammation of the membranes that cover the brain. A CT scan and evaluation of spinal fluid (obtained via a spinal tap, in which fluid is drawn from the lower back region of the spine) can confirm or rule out this diagnosis.
A headache accompanied by neurological impairment (for example, difficulty speaking or walking, weakness of one side of the body, or double vision)	Brain tumor, stroke, or abscess. Imaging tests, such as a CT or MRI scan, are required to evaluate the situation.
A headache that feels like a blow to the head (also known as thunderclap headache)	Bleeding around the brain. A CT scan and a spinal tap are necessary to make a diagnosis.
A headache that slowly but relentlessly gets worse over weeks or months	Brain tumor. Evaluation by a CT or MRI scan may be needed.
A headache with constant, severe, throbbing pain in the temple region, particularly in people over age 60	Temporal arteritis (see "When it hurts to the touch: Temporal arteritis," page 6). Blood tests and a biopsy are needed to confirm the diagnosis.
A headache that occurs frequently, if not daily, especially in the back of the head or neck, is present on awakening, and improves when you get out of bed	High spinal fluid pressure.

- a headache with confusion or loss of consciousness
- a headache along with pain in the eye or ear
- a relentless headache when you were previously headache-free
- a headache that is incapacitating.

Table 1 (see page 4) explains what these might mean. Note that you should always take children who have recurring headaches to the doctor, especially when the pain occurs at night or is present when the child wakes in the morning. Under rare circumstances, this might indicate a brain tumor.

The office visit

Your physician will try to determine the causes of your headaches and design a treatment plan. Expect some detailed questions about your headaches (see "What your doctor will want to know," at right) and possibly some basic laboratory tests.

He or she will perform a physical exam, including a blood pressure check and a careful look inside your eyes with an ophthalmoscope. Increased pressure in the head, which can be a sign of a brain tumor, can cause swelling of the optic nerve; the ophthalmoscope examination can reveal such swelling. In some people, tension and migraine headaches produce telltale signs such as spasms in the neck and shoulder muscles and tender areas—known as "trigger spots"—at the back of the head; your doctor may check for these. Your doctor might also examine how your jaw functions, as headaches can be a sign of temporomandibular joint (TMJ) disorder. But in most people who have tension or migraine headaches, the physical examination doesn't turn up anything unusual—which is good.

That's why an accurate, detailed description of your symptoms is invaluable to your physician. Note when your headaches begin; what they feel like; particular situations that prompt or worsen them; and the location, frequency, intensity, and duration of the pain. It may help to keep a headache diary (see the form on page 7 and "Keeping a headache diary," page 8).

Your physician will also want to know about other symptoms linked to your headaches, what's helped relieve your pain in the past, which nonprescription and prescription medications you currently take, and whether other family members have

▶ What your doctor will want to know

Because common headaches have few, if any, measurable effects on the body, tests aren't likely to turn up much in the way of helpful information. Instead, your doctor will rely on the information you provide about your pain. Before an appointment, you may find it useful to jot down the answers to these questions:
- When did your headaches begin?
- Does anything seem related to their onset?
- How often do they occur?
- How long do they last?
- When do they occur?
- Where is the pain located?
- How severe is it?
- What does it feel like?
- Do you notice any other symptoms before or during the headaches?
- Does anything trigger or worsen the headaches?
- Does anything ease the pain?
- Does anyone in your family have a history of headaches?
- How is your family and work life?
- How have the headaches affected your life?

experienced problem headaches. A broad discussion about your life, focusing on stresses at home or work and the impact of your headaches, can also help your doctor reach the correct diagnosis and plan the best treatment.

Anyone over age 40 who's bothered by headaches should also schedule an appointment with an ophthalmologist. Because eyestrain or squinting can cause headaches, a thorough eye exam may reveal that something as simple as getting new glasses might alleviate your pain. However, a more serious problem could also be at fault. Glaucoma, a condition marked by elevated pressure inside the eye, can cause headache-like pain around the eyes or forehead. Glaucoma is treatable, but it can lead to blindness if it goes undetected or untreated for many years. Acute closed-angle glaucoma, in which pressure rises rapidly inside the eye, is a medical emergency and should be treated right away. Symptoms include pain, blurred vision, and sometimes halos (colored rings around lights).

Diagnostic tests

Headaches don't always match their textbook descriptions. For example, you may experience symptoms of different types of headaches at the same time, and there is no definitive test to determine which type you have. A headache produced by stress or tight muscles can resemble one caused by an underlying disease. To exclude more serious causes, your doctor may perform tests that show the body's internal structures, such as a computed tomography (CT) scan or a magnetic resonance imaging (MRI) scan.

Considering how many people get headaches—and how long the list of potential causes is—remarkably few people need special testing. No tests are needed for obvious tension or migraine headaches, for example. However, doctors sometimes recommend a CT scan to help diagnose sinus headaches, since imaging can reveal sinus blockage.

If you've had headaches that haven't changed much in intensity or frequency over the years, you're less likely to need additional tests than someone who is just starting to experience headaches or someone whose headaches have gotten worse. If you have pain that occurs consistently in the same location or on one side of the head—both of which could result from an underlying medical condition, such as a tumor or a blood vessel abnormality (see "When it hurts to the touch: Temporal arteritis," below)—your doctor may order additional tests. On the other hand, a headache that regularly shifts from one side to the other may not need further evaluation, since this suggests a less ominous cause such as migraines.

CT scan

A CT scan is taken with a special x-ray machine. Rather than sending one wide x-ray beam through your body, this machine sends out many beams from

continued on page 8

When it hurts to the touch: Temporal arteritis

A severe, constant headache may be one of the first signs of temporal arteritis, a condition caused by inflammation of the large temporal arteries located on either side of the head. Also known as cranial or giant-cell arteritis, this painful condition is twice as common in women as in men and usually occurs in people ages 50 or older.

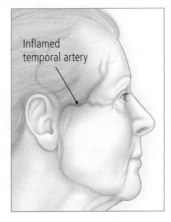

Inflamed temporal artery

People with temporal arteritis describe the pain as severe, throbbing, and burning—most often at the temple on one side of the head. Other symptoms, such as a low-grade fever, fatigue, loss of weight or appetite, or a tender scalp or temple may also occur. Chewing may cause aching in the jaw muscles. If you suspect a headache may be caused by temporal arteritis, seek a medical evaluation as soon as possible.

Doctors don't know what triggers the problem, but it involves a misguided immune response in which antibodies attack the blood vessel walls. The resulting swelling can progressively narrow the affected vessels, reducing blood flow. In severe cases, arteries become totally blocked. If this happens in the artery supplying the retina, it threatens the vision in that eye. If an artery that serves the brain is impaired, a stroke could result. However, when caught and treated early, temporal arteritis responds well to medication.

A doctor who suspects temporal arteritis will check your blood's sedimentation rate. This simple blood test measures the rate at which your red blood cells settle to the bottom of a test tube. A rate that's higher than normal suggests there's inflammation in your body. The only sure way to diagnose the condition, however, is to remove part of the blood vessel and examine it under a microscope for changes in the artery wall.

Confirming temporal arteritis with a biopsy is crucial because the condition requires long-term treatment with drugs called steroids, which reduce inflammation. Your doctor will want to be sure the diagnosis is correct before prescribing steroids for an extended period. Your doctor may even begin steroid therapy as a precautionary measure before taking the blood vessel biopsy. If your doctor does prescribe a steroid, such as prednisone, you will probably need to take it until all symptoms have disappeared and the results of further laboratory tests are normal. This usually takes at least a month. The dosage is then gradually decreased. Some physicians believe continuing low-dose steroids for a year or two may prevent recurrences.

Headache diary

Your doctor may ask you to keep a headache diary to help pinpoint triggers and patterns of your headaches. Start by noting the date of any headache you experience. In addition, pay close attention to the other items in the list—the times your headache began and ended, any warning signs, and so forth—and record this information as well.

Note: Permission is granted to reproduce this page of the report for individual use. You can also download copies from www.health.harvard.edu/headache-diary.

	FIRST EPISODE	SECOND EPISODE	THIRD EPISODE
Date/day of the week of headache			
Time of onset			
Time of resolution			
Warning signs			
Location(s) of the pain			
Type of pain			
Intensity of the pain (on a scale from 1 to 10)			
Additional symptoms			
Activities/circumstances at time of onset			
Time of most recent meal prior to onset			
Food/drink most recently consumed prior to onset			
Medication(s) taken for headache			
Response to medication(s)			
Other action(s) taken for relief			
Response to action(s)			
Last menstrual period (start and end dates)			
Medication(s) currently taken for other condition(s)			

continued from page 6
many angles. A computer uses the results to generate detailed, cross-sectional pictures of your body. In some cases, a contrast dye is administered intravenously to define the brain structures more clearly.

The CT scan provides a much clearer picture of your head than a regular x-ray. The test is painless and can help identify tumors, bleeding, areas of damaged brain tissue, and even sinus infections. However, these scans expose you to far more radiation than a conventional x-ray and should be avoided when possible.

The test takes only a few minutes.

MRI scan

Although MRI creates an image similar to that produced by a CT scan, the technique is quite different. Rather than using x-rays, the MRI machine relies on a strong magnetic field. Tissues give off minute electromagnetic waves in frequencies that differ according to the type of tissue involved. A computer tallies the vibrations and uses this information to create cross-sectional images on many different planes. These remarkably detailed pictures can show the difference between brain tissue and tumors and highlight areas of the brain that have been damaged by a stroke or other neurological conditions.

For an MRI scan, you must lie motionless inside a large tube located in the center of a room-sized machine. The scanning process is noisy, so you must wear ear protection. Some people feel claustrophobic inside the device, but many testing facilities provide earphones so you can listen to music to ease some of the anxiety. MRI machines of a more open design are available in some facilities. The procedure takes 20 to 45 minutes. If intravenous dye is needed to enhance the image, it's usually given halfway through the procedure.

Keeping a headache diary

A headache diary can be valuable in helping you and your doctor diagnose and treat your headaches. You can use it to map out the characteristics of your headaches, including their frequency, duration, and intensity. It can also help in identifying possible triggers and related symptoms, as well as tracking the dosage and effectiveness of any medications you're taking.

There are many ways to keep a headache diary. You can use a preprinted form like the one on page 7 of this report, or use a regular calendar or notebook to record this information. Alternatively, you can download a headache app for your computer, tablet, or smartphone.

Your doctor may recommend keeping such a diary every day for a week, a month, or the duration of your treatment. He or she may review the diary with you to assess your progress, weigh the effectiveness of medications, or make adjustments in your treatment plan. ♥

Tension headaches

Tension headaches (officially known as "tension-type headaches") are the most common type of headache, affecting most people at some point in their lives. These include the typical mild, intermittent, easy-to-treat headaches that many of us experience. Although most people have them only occasionally, a small percentage of individuals suffer from tension headaches on a more regular basis. Tension headaches can occur weekly or even daily or near-daily (see "Chronic headaches," page 33).

The term "tension headache" is somewhat misleading, suggesting that it results solely from being tense. While physical and emotional stress often play a role in these headaches, especially occasional ones, tension is only one of the factors that can precipitate a tension headache. For chronic tension headaches, the causes can include things like illness, surgery, and head or neck injuries. What's more, some of the triggers for tension headaches—such as missed meals or lack of sleep—overlap with those of migraines, suggesting that the two headache types may share some of the same underlying causes, including genetic predisposition. Unlike migraine headaches, however, tension headaches are not accompanied by other symptoms, such as nausea, vomiting, or blurred vision. Nor have researchers linked them to other migraine triggers, such as foods and hormonal changes.

Tension headaches are common at any age, but women are more susceptible, as is true for headaches in general. These headaches usually strike in the afternoon, causing mild or moderate pain. However, people with a lesser-known type of tension headache caused by a temporomandibular joint (TMJ) disorder may experience morning headaches (see "Tense jaw joints: A source of some tension headaches," page 10).

The pain of a tension headache may envelop your entire head or be limited to one portion of it, such as your forehead or the back or top of your head. Many people describe the sensation as a dull tightness or pressure that occurs in a bandlike pattern (see Figure 1, below). The intensity of the pain may fluctuate, but it shouldn't be intense enough to keep you from functioning during the day or sleeping at night.

Triggers and aggravators

In some cases, the pain of a tension headache is caused by tightness in the muscles of the scalp and the back of the neck, which can be triggered by a variety of emotional and physical factors. A survey published in the journal *Headache* reported that stress was the most common factor precipitating tension headaches.

Other frequent triggers (in order of their prevalence) included missed meals, lack of sleep, and fatigue.

Figure 1: Tension headache pain

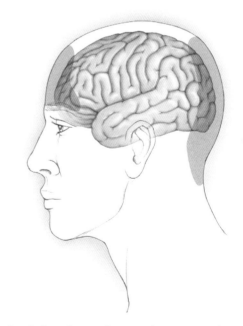

Tension headaches often produce steady pain across the forehead or in the back of the head. Sometimes your entire head hurts, with a sensation often described as a dull tightness.

Physical problems, such as eyestrain, whiplash, or poor posture, can also act as triggers. In addition to triggering tension headaches, these problems can aggravate an existing tension headache.

Relieving tension headaches

Most intermittent tension headaches—the regular, mild headaches you might experience from time to time—can be easily managed with an over-the-counter (OTC) painkiller such as ibuprofen, without requiring medical care.

However, OTC painkillers and even stronger prescription pain relievers may not fully relieve tension headaches, and they may actually worsen the situation by turning an occasional problem into a chronic one. That's because both OTC and prescription pain relievers target only the symptom of tension headaches (pain), without addressing the underlying cause. If your headaches are caused by a problem like chronic muscle tightness, then relying too much on pain relievers may cause "rebound" headaches that gradually increase in frequency. To make matters worse, frequent use of pain relievers (more than two days a week), especially pills containing caffeine, may make other medications less effective at relieving your tension headaches (see "Medication overuse headaches," page 33). That's why targeting the underlying cause is a better strategy for more severe or recurring tension headaches (see "Preventing tension head-

Tense jaw joints: A source of some tension headaches

If you wake up in the morning with a dull, deep headache (which may or not subside during the day), it may stem from a temporomandibular joint (TMJ) disorder—that is, a disorder in the jaw joints. These flexible joints, found on each side of the head just in front of the ear, connect the temporal bone of the skull to the lower jaw, or mandible (hence, "temporomandibular"). A cushioning disc, or articular disc (see illustration), allows smooth movement of this joint. However, whiplash or a heavy blow to the jaw can trigger TMJ disorder, which leads to tenderness in the face, jaw joint area, neck, and shoulders, as well as in or around the ear when you chew, speak, or open your mouth wide.

Another common cause of TMJ disorder is tooth grinding and clenching, a condition known as bruxism that occurs in about one in 20 adults. People who grind their teeth during sleep usually rub their lower teeth against their upper teeth in a back-and-forth or side-to-side motion, creating a noise that sounds like chewing on hard crackers or ice cubes. Clenching (which can happen during sleep or while you're awake) is more like a rocking motion of the lower teeth against the uppers. Some people don't realize they have bruxism unless a bed partner mentions it or a dentist points out worn-down areas on the teeth. Most people with bruxism don't develop TMJ disorder, but frequent grinders can develop stiff neck muscles—another possible trigger for tension headaches. The pain of these headaches usually centers around the sides and back of the head.

Other symptoms of a TMJ disorder include a clicking or popping of the jaw joints, pain in or around the jaws, and locking or limited opening of your mouth. If you think your headaches might be due to bruxism or TMJ disorder, consult your dentist, who may refer you to an orofacial or craniofacial pain specialist (also see "Resources," page 38). For some people, a dental night guard—a small piece of hard plastic custom-fitted to your upper teeth—will help reduce the symptoms of bruxism. Some people need to wear specialized mouth guards during the day, and many benefit from stress management (see "A prescription for stress relief," page 31, and "Physical therapy, massage, chiropractic, osteopathy," page 32). In rare cases, people need surgery to correct a damaged joint.

Temporalis muscle

Temporal bone

Temporomandibular joint

Articular disc

Masseter muscle

Mandible (jaw)

MedicusMedia.com

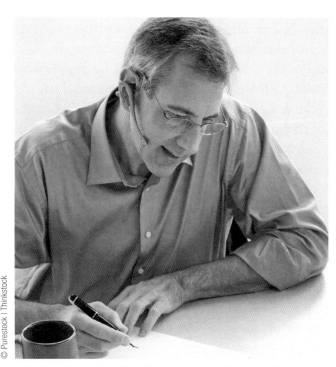
A headset for your landline phone or earbuds for your cellphone can help you avoid awkward positions that strain your neck and cause stiff muscles.

aches," at right). A fast-acting but short-lived muscle relaxant such as carisoprodol (Soma, Vanadom) or metaxalone (Skelaxin) can counter tightness in head and neck muscles. While these medications don't relieve pain any more effectively than OTC painkillers, they do address the underlying cause of the tension headache. Despite their name, these drugs don't directly relax tense muscles. Instead, they slow the functioning of your central nervous system, creating an overall calming effect. They work quickly, taking effect within 15 to 30 minutes, but the effects last only three to four hours. Still, such medications typically outlast the usual tension headache, which rarely continues for more than a few hours.

Unlike some muscle relaxants, carisoprodol and metaxalone generally don't produce tolerance (the need for increasingly larger doses to obtain the same effect), but they may cause drowsiness and fatigue, which, in turn, can impair mental and physical functioning. Thus, avoid driving, operating heavy equipment, or performing other hazardous tasks while taking these medications. Muscle relaxants aren't recommended for people with liver or kidney disease or a history of drug dependency.

Preventing tension headaches

If you have frequent tension headaches (more often than once or twice a week), finding a helpful prevention strategy is vital, so you don't become overly reliant on painkillers or muscle relaxants. Doctors often advise people with tension headaches not to skip meals, to get enough sleep, and to pace themselves to avoid becoming overly tired. You might also consider trying acupuncture or rubbing peppermint oil on your temples (see the Special Section, "Self-help and alternative strategies to ease headache pain," page 27). Other options include relaxation strategies, trigger point injections, and medications.

In addition, you should try not to subject your head and neck muscles to prolonged strain. The following tips may help.

- If you sit for lengthy periods of time in front of a computer, try changing your position every so often. Frequent, brief breaks can help you avoid awkward positions that predispose your neck and shoulder muscles to tensing. Simply walking across the room or shrugging your shoulders and bending your neck can get the kinks out.
- Position the top of your computer monitor just below eye level, so you don't have to tilt your head down to work on it.
- Limit tablet time. A 2015 study found that when you look down at a tablet in your lap, your neck muscles work three to five times harder than they would if you were looking straight ahead.
- Don't rest your chin on your chest while reading.
- Avoid cupping the telephone between your shoulder and ear. If you use the telephone often, you may want to buy a headset.
- Avoid excessive gum-chewing, which can strain jaw muscles.
- Try not to clench your jaw or grind your teeth.
- Apply a heating pad to the back of the neck and shoulders for 15 to 20 minutes at the end of each day.

Relaxation strategies

Various types of relaxation therapies—either physical approaches or mind-body techniques—prevent tension headaches, although these work only if you practice them on a regular basis, preferably every day.

The simplest strategy is to apply a heating pad to your neck and shoulders to relax the muscles when they feel tight. Exercising these muscles also helps, by strengthening and stretching them. Your doctor may be able to provide examples of suitable exercises or a referral to a physical therapist. Other physical techniques to relieve tension headaches include massage to relax muscles or traction to stretch them.

Two types of mind-body relaxation therapies may also be useful.

- Autogenic training is a technique in which you learn to focus your attention on various parts of your body, in succession, and then imagine them becoming warm and heavy in order to relax them.
- Biofeedback is another technique, in which you learn to recognize when your muscles are becoming tense and learn how to relax them, based on signals from your own body. In biofeedback for tension headaches, typically a therapist will attach electrodes to your skin to detect electrical signals from your neck and shoulder muscles. When you become tense, the biofeedback machine may beep or flash a light. Eventually, even when you're not hooked up to the machine, you recognize when you are becoming tense, and you find ways to relax the muscles before they tighten so much you develop a tension headache.

Medications to prevent tension headaches

The tricyclic medications amitriptyline (Elavil, Endep) and doxepin (Adapin, Sinequan) have proved most effective for preventing tension headaches. One study found that three out of four people taking daily ami-

triptyline reported significant improvement in their head pain. Because they cause drowsiness, tricyclic medications are particularly useful for people who have both tension headaches and insomnia. If one tricyclic drug isn't effective, another may work. Changing the dosage can also help (see "Tricyclics," page 20).

A long-acting muscle relaxant, such as cyclobenzaprine (Flexeril) or tizanidine (Zanaflex), can also stave off tension headaches. Like their fast-acting relatives, these drugs slow the central nervous system, indirectly relaxing tense muscles. They also have similar side effects, including drowsiness and fatigue. Unlike carisoprodol or metaxalone, these drugs take an hour or so to work; however, their effects can last as long as a day. To reduce the likelihood that side effects will disrupt your routine, you should take cyclobenzaprine or tizanidine only once daily, before bedtime.

Trigger point injections

Some people with tension headaches have very sensitive areas, known as trigger points, at the back of the neck or shoulders. Touching these tender areas sometimes prompts a headache. If your doctor identifies such trigger points during the physical examination and other treatments fail to provide relief, injecting a local anesthetic into these areas may eliminate the pain and prevent the headache from occurring again. In most cases, you'll get a few days of relief from an injection that's typically given every two to three weeks on an ongoing or as-needed basis. This option has limitations, though. First, you must receive the shot at a clinic, hospital, or your doctor's office. Second, many people are uneasy about receiving a shot in the neck or shoulders. ♥

Sinus headaches

Sinus headaches are another common form of headache. The sinuses are air-filled spaces above, between, and beneath your eyes, flanking your nose. They serve several functions, including warming and moistening the air you breathe and lightening the weight of the head. Both the nose and sinuses are lined with a thin membrane that swells and produces mucus in response to irritation. Normally, the mucus from the sinuses drains through small openings, known as ostia, which connect the sinuses to the nasal passages.

Sinus headaches can occur in three situations: when the inner membrane becomes inflamed, when fluid builds up in the sinuses and can't drain out through the nose, or when pressure in the sinuses is lower than environmental air pressure (sometimes called barometric pressure because it is measured by an instrument known as a barometer). Whatever the cause, sinus headache pain is most often felt in the center of the face, the bridge of the nose, and the cheeks (see Figure 2, at right). It may also occur behind the eyes or in the center of the forehead and be accompanied by nasal congestion and clear or opaque nasal discharge.

How sinus headaches develop

Any condition that causes the nose or sinus membranes to become swollen can narrow or completely block the ostia, resulting in a sinus headache.

Inflammation of the nose and sinus membranes, known as rhinosinusitis, is usually triggered by allergy or viral infection. Less often, rhinosinusitis is caused by exposure to secondhand smoke, perfume, or other inhaled chemicals.

Sometimes, particularly when the inflammation is sufficient to block drainage from the sinuses, bacteria that normally live in the sinuses take advantage of the situation, producing a bacterial infection. A bacterial sinus infection not only causes head pain, but also often produces foul-smelling, yellow-green discharge,

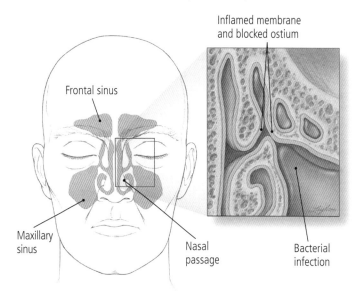

Figure 2: Sinus infection (sinusitis)

Inflamed membrane and blocked ostium

Frontal sinus

Maxillary sinus

Nasal passage

Bacterial infection

Normally, mucus drains from the sinuses into the nasal passages through small openings, known as ostia. But these openings can become blocked from allergy, viral infection, or some other cause. This congestion can lead to a bacterial sinus infection, which is often accompanied by yellow or green nasal discharge, a bad taste in the mouth, and sometimes fever.

sometimes coughed up from the back of the throat, that can leave a bad taste in the mouth. A bacterial infection can also cause fever, and, at its worst, chills and uncontrollable shaking.

Air pressure inside the sinuses also contributes to sinus headaches. Typically, the air pressure inside the sinuses is the same as the pressure in the nose and in the air around you. But blockage of the ostia can result in unusually low air pressure inside the sinuses, which produces sinus pain.

Managing sinus headaches

Treating sinus headaches usually involves over-the-counter (OTC) medications that reduce inflammation in the sinuses and obstruction of the ostia.

An antihistamine blocks the action of histamine (a substance released during an allergic reaction that causes mucosal swelling and mucus production). Antihistamines are particularly effective if the sinus headache is triggered by allergies, and many are available over the counter.

Antihistamines often have side effects—in particular, drowsiness, slowed reaction time, impaired judgment, and nasal dryness. Older "first-generation" antihistamines—in particular, diphenhydramine (Benadryl), clemastine (Tavist), and brompheniramine (an ingredient in the combination product Dimetapp)—are more likely to cause such effects. Another older antihistamine, chlorpheniramine (Chlor-Trimeton, others), is less sedating, though it still causes drowsiness in about 10% of users. A newer generation of antihistamines, also available over the counter, minimize such side effects. These newer antihistamines include loratadine (Claritin, Alavert, others) and cetirizine (Zyrtec).

You can also try guaifenesin, an OTC medication that thins the mucus so that it drains more easily. (Mucinex is especially effective.) Another option is a decongestant, which also reduces swelling and opens up the nasal and sinus passages. Decongestants can be helpful when a sinus headache is the result of changes in barometric pressure. Such medications, or a steam bath, will usually do the trick. Some experts recommend the use of a neti pot or other system for rinsing the sinuses, despite a small risk of using tainted water.

Saline nasal sprays can also help clear congested sinuses. Medicated nasal sprays, however, are remarkably dependence-inducing and should not be used more than a few days at a time, because the congestion can rebound, leading to a vicious cycle of treatment and further congestion.

If you have chronic allergies, your doctor may recommend one of several antihistamines available only by prescription, which come in pill or spray forms, or a corticosteroid nasal spray.

Is it a sinus headache or a migraine?

Migraine headaches are often mistaken for sinus headaches; in fact, 86% or more of patients who suspect that they have sinus headaches in fact have migraines. Why the confusion?

Migraines and sinus headaches share some symptoms, including pressure in the face, an association with changes in barometric pressure or seasonal weather, and dysfunction of the autonomic nervous system, which controls many of the involuntary functions in your body, including heart rate, blood pressure, and sweating. In the case of migraines, autonomic dysfunction can cause eye redness, eyelid swelling or drooping, tear production, sinus congestion, and even a runny nose.

The mistake can be perpetuated if a doctor prescribes an antibiotic and steroids for a suspected sinus infection and the migraine headache gets better. The improvement is caused by a few factors. Steroids can help relieve migraine pain, and antibiotics can have a powerful placebo effect. Alternatively, the headache may go away on its own, but you may ascribe the relief to medications. A correct diagnosis is important, as the cycle of treating migraines as sinus infections can lead to unnecessary overuse of steroids and antibiotics.

A sinus headache due to an infection can often be distinguished from a migraine by the presence of thick, green or yellow mucus and a fever. If an imaging study or evaluation with an endoscope looking up the nose shows a sinus problem, then the headaches are likely related to that, unless they continue after the sinus problem is successfully treated.

Yellow or green sinus discharge in the back of your throat sometimes means you have a bacterial infection, which warrants a call to your doctor. You'll need an antibiotic and a decongestant or steroid nasal spray to treat this condition. To confirm a diagnosis, your doctor may order some tests, such as a CT scan, although the use of imaging is generally restricted to people with recurrent sinus infections and those with symptoms that don't respond to treatment. If you develop high fever, severe pain, or chills and uncontrollable shaking, contact your doctor immediately. ♥

Migraine headaches

Migraine pain has been called indescribable, yet 35 million Americans know it all too well. Horror author Stephen King, himself a migraineur (someone who suffers from migraines), penned a vivid description of a migraine in his novel *Firestarter*:

The headache would get worse until it was a smashing weight, sending red pain through his head and neck with every pulse beat. Bright lights would make his eyes water helplessly and send darts of agony into the flesh just behind his eyes. Small noises magnified, ordinary noises insupportable. The headache would worsen until it felt as if his head were being crushed inside an inquisitor's lovecap …. He would be next to helpless.

King doesn't describe the pattern of the pain, but the word "migraine" itself tells you something about that. It is the French derivation of the Greek word *hemikrania*, meaning "half a head," since migraine

fastfact | Approximately 10% to 15% of the adult population—one in five women and one in 20 men— have migraines.

pain usually affects only one side of the head, most often at the temple (see Figure 3, below left). Migraine pain ranges from moderate to severe, and the side of the head that's affected can vary from one attack to the next, or even during a single episode. Unlike tension headaches, migraines can keep you from functioning or sleeping, and they can even rouse you from sound slumber. Most people describe the pain as throbbing. It can also be sharp, almost as if a dagger is piercing your temple or eye.

Tense head, neck, and shoulder muscles can accompany a migraine headache. In fact, measurements of muscle tension tend to be higher in migraine sufferers than in people with tension headaches. In most cases, this is thought to be an involuntary response to the pain, rather than its cause, although tight muscles can also trigger a migraine headache. Bright lights and loud noises worsen the pain and may prompt someone with a migraine headache to seek out quiet, dimly lit places. Nausea and vomiting are common during a migraine; odors may aggravate these symptoms.

People who suffer from frequent or even daily migraines (chronic migraines) also are more likely to have additional health concerns, such as anxiety, depression, insomnia, irritable bowel syndrome, or restless legs syndrome. Addressing these other problems—or comorbidities, as they're known medically—is an important aspect of optimal migraine treatment.

Anatomy of an attack

To most people, "migraine" refers only to a particular type of head pain. Actually, the term encompasses a broader set of changes that may occur throughout the

---

Figure 3: Migraine headache pain

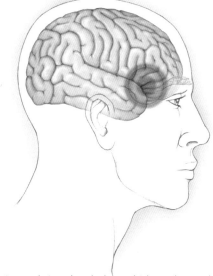

Unlike tension and sinus headaches, which produce a dull, steady pain, the pain of migraine headache is throbbing or sharp. It usually occurs on one side of the head only, confined to the temple, eye, or back of the head.

body, although not all of these symptoms are evident in every person who has migraine.

Typically, the early sensations include a change in mood, appetite, or activity level. These symptoms, known as prodromal symptoms or the prodrome, warn you that a migraine headache is on the way.

Some people also experience visual disturbances shortly before the migraine begins. These might include seeing sparkling or flashing zigzag lines (scintillations) or blank spots (scotomas; see Figure 4, below). Less often, people will experience tingling on one side of the body, often in the hand, arm, and face. Such visual and sensory disturbances generally last anywhere from 10 to 30 minutes and are known as auras. The presence or absence of an aura determines whether an episode is a classic migraine (with an aura) or common migraine (without an aura).

What causes a migraine headache and—when it occurs—an aura? Experts aren't sure (see Figure 5, page 17). For many years, scientists believed that a tightening of the brain arteries interfered with blood flow. The arteries would then dilate to compensate, not only in the brain but also outside the brain, where the dilation can cause nerve fibers to release inflammatory compounds. Although scientists still believe that this combination of blood vessel dilation and

inflammation causes migraines, they no longer think that the tightening of cerebral arteries underlies the aura.

Here's why: although researchers have confirmed that the aura coincides with a reduction in brain blood flow, this reduction is milder than would be seen with blood vessel constriction or spasm. Instead, many experts now suspect that the migraine aura is produced by a phenomenon known as spreading depression, which is a wave of decreased electrical activity (indicating lower brain cell functioning) and diminished blood flow that inexplicably passes across the cerebral cortex. As nerve cell activity is suppressed, cerebral blood flow diminishes. The areas of lowered activity gradually spread, as if washing across the brain, causing the symptoms of an aura.

The altered cerebral blood flow and electrical activity occur first in the primary visual cortex, which may help explain why visual disturbances often accompany the aura. Symptoms affecting the extremities, such as numbness and tingling, may occur when the spreading depression reaches a part of the brain known as the primary sensorimotor cortex. The spreading depression usually stops about halfway across the brain. At that point, a parallel process, involving a combination of blood vessel dilation and inflammation, may

Figure 4: The visual aura of a migraine: Scintillating scotoma

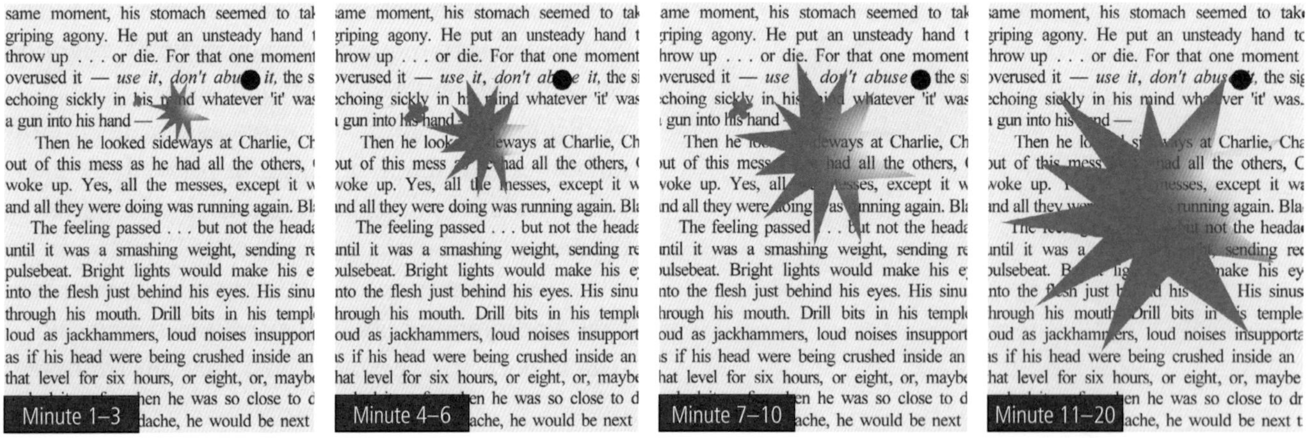

Minute 1–3   Minute 4–6   Minute 7–10   Minute 11–20

Migraine auras often include a blind spot or area in one side of the field of vision, known as a scotoma. Although scotomas usually appear black in people with other conditions, in migraines they are typically white or gray, or, in rare cases, colored. The scotoma typically appears as a shimmering zigzag in the shape of a crescent that expands across one side of a person's field of vision. The above drawing shows what a person experiencing this phenomenon might see while reading a book. Visual auras typically last about 20 minutes and are often but not always followed by a headache and the other typical features of migraine.

Figure 5: Three theories about the cause of migraines

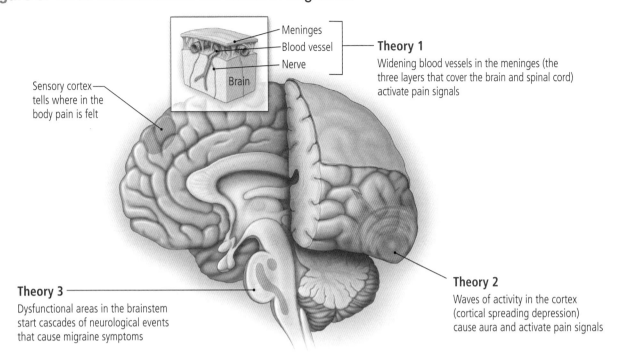

Meninges
Blood vessel
Nerve
Brain

Theory 1
Widening blood vessels in the meninges (the three layers that cover the brain and spinal cord) activate pain signals

Sensory cortex tells where in the body pain is felt

Theory 3
Dysfunctional areas in the brainstem start cascades of neurological events that cause migraine symptoms

Theory 2
Waves of activity in the cortex (cortical spreading depression) cause aura and activate pain signals

be causing headache pain. Bolstering this theory is the fact that a resting brain is more susceptible to spreading depression than an active one, which may explain why migraine attacks often strike as people unwind after a stressful period.

A migraine attack can also consist of an aura only, with no subsequent headache. This type of migraine is more common in older people and is sometimes confused with a transient ischemic attack (TIA), also called a ministroke, which often is the first sign of an impending stroke. TIAs occur when a blood clot temporarily interrupts blood flow through one of the smaller arteries in the brain. Symptoms may include weakness on one side of the body or blindness in one eye or one side of the visual field. If you've suffered from migraines throughout your life, remember these similarities, because you may be able to avoid expensive and sometimes risky tests for TIAs. But if in doubt, err on the side of caution.

Timing of attacks

Many migraine attacks occur in the evening or at night and, ironically, may be the result of the body's attempt to relax after the day's stresses. Blood vessels tighten in response to stress and widen during relaxation, and dilated blood vessels in the head are a chief trigger for migraine pain. What's more, relaxation lowers an individual's pain threshold. Thus, an evening or nighttime migraine usually occurs after a particularly intense day or a period of prolonged stress.

Both the frequency and the duration of migraine headaches vary from person to person. Migraine headaches usually last at least four hours and no longer than 24 hours, although they can leave a lingering pain that persists for days or even longer. On occasion, however, the migraine itself can last for days, especially in women who have these headaches before or during menstruation.

Who's at risk?

During childhood, migraines affect boys and girls equally. But after puberty, the situation shifts, with women more likely to experience migraine headaches. About 9% of men and 16% of women suffer from migraine headaches. The tendency for migraines runs in families. These headaches also seem to be connected with motion sickness, as many adult migraine sufferers recall bouts of carsickness as children.

Figure 6: Menstrual migraine

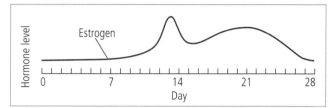

Most migraine headaches in women occur when estrogen levels are low or falling—usually right before a period starts (days 27 to 28 of the cycle) and during menstruation (days 0 to 4 or 5), but sometimes also around the time of ovulation (day 14), when estrogen levels begin to fall rapidly from their peak.

Estrogens have long been linked to headaches, but the reasons behind this association remain elusive. Women are more likely to experience migraines and other kinds of headaches around the time of menstruation and, to a lesser extent, ovulation (see Figure 6, above). Migraine headaches that occur in the days before menstruation tend to be particularly severe and incapacitating. (At menopause, menstrual migraine headaches should improve as long as you don't take hormone therapy—which may actually increase the frequency and intensity of the attacks.)

Starting or stopping estrogen-containing medications can also trigger migraines. Birth control pills may increase the frequency or intensity of attacks—usually during the placebo week when the pills don't contain any estrogen. By contrast, low-estrogen birth control pills that are taken continuously may prevent menstrual migraine headaches in some women.

Migraine triggers

Many factors that cause tension headaches—such as stress, lack of sleep, or missing a meal—can also trigger migraine headaches (see "Common triggers," at right). Migraine sufferers seem to be overly sensitive to sensory stimuli; however, the specific stimuli that trigger a headache vary widely from person to person. Studies on migraine and diet have cast doubt on the common idea that certain foods consistently cause migraines, and doctors are relying less and less on prescribing specific "migraine diets." However, on an individual basis, people often find that alcohol or a particular food or additive may prompt an attack (see "Migraines and food," page 19).

Of course, if you can identify such a trigger, your prevention strategy is simple: try to avoid it. However, most migraineurs have dozens of triggers, and it's often impossible to avoid all of them. What's more, the effect of a given trigger on your headache can be unpredictable. But to your advantage, it often takes more than one trigger to cause a migraine. For example, stress might not cause an attack without fatigue. In such a case, you may be able to use your list of triggers to manage a headache, if not prevent it. If a woman knows she's more vulnerable to migraines during menstruation, she may want to avoid alcohol during this time, given that a migraine can be triggered by just a glass or two of wine. Migraine headaches are also most common on weekends, perhaps because people are more likely to drink alcohol, sleep too little, oversleep in the morning, or experience caffeine withdrawal (some people drink less coffee on weekends or have their first cup later than usual). When migraine headaches are frequent, they can cause muscle tightness, which can, in turn, trigger more headaches.

How does a trigger spur a migraine headache? Experts don't know for sure whether it first causes dilation or inflammation of blood vessels. There are staunch partisans for each view. Indeed, different triggers may work through different mechanisms. The two processes also seem interconnected, and their interaction may foster a migraine headache once it's started. For instance, widening of a blood vessel causes inflammation, and inflammation causes a blood vessel to expand. Researchers believe that different triggers affect this relationship in different ways.

▶ Common triggers

People with migraine headaches cite the following as the top five headache triggers:

1. stress or tension
2. missing meals
3. fatigue
4. lack of sleep
5. smoke or some sort of odor.

Migraines and food

There's no one "migraine diet" that works for everyone, but these are some of the foods most commonly reported to trigger migraines:

- alcoholic beverages
- avocados
- bananas

- beans (except green or wax)
- caffeinated beverages (tea, coffee, cola, etc.)
- cheeses, aged and unpasteurized (Brie, Camembert, Cheddar, Gruyere, Stilton, etc.)
- chicken livers
- chocolate

- citrus fruits
- fermented, pickled, or marinated foods
- herring
- monosodium glutamate (MSG)
- nitrates (found in cured meats)

- nuts and peanut butter
- onions
- peas
- pork
- sour cream
- vinegar (except white)
- yogurt.

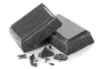

While avoiding triggers is important, it doesn't mean you should live in fear of every potential trigger, especially those you might otherwise enjoy. Instead, experts say it's worth trying to find out what truly triggers a migraine for you. A good way to do this is by keeping a headache diary (see page 8).

Preventing migraine headaches

When migraine attacks are particularly severe, do not respond to treatment, or occur more than three or four times a month, it's time to look into preventive strategies. In addition to identifying and avoiding triggers, preventive approaches include a procedure called transcutaneous electrical nerve stimulation (TENS), various drugs, and alternative treatments (especially acupuncture; see page 31).

Transcutaneous electrical nerve stimulation

Using electricity to stimulate the nerves is a common way to manage chronic pain throughout the body. But scientists have only recently begun to apply this technology, which is called transcutaneous electrical nerve stimulation (TENS), to migraines. It's not clear how TENS works against migraines. According to one hypothesis, it disrupts electrical patterns in the brain in ways that raise the so-called migraine threshold.

The first TENS device for migraine prevention was approved by the FDA in 2014. Cefaly (the trade name of the device) is a battery-powered electrode mounted on a plastic headband. It can be used at home as needed when a headache strikes, or daily as a preventive treatment. Placed directly on the forehead, it applies a current that stimulates branches of nerves in the brainstem that process pain. During the study that led to its approval, migraineurs using Cefaly reported a significant drop in the average number of headache days per month—from seven days to five. However, it takes time for the device to become effective, and most participants didn't report a benefit until the study's third month.

Beta blockers

Doctors have prescribed these medications for years to treat high blood pressure, abnormal heart rhythms, and angina. Beta blockers may relieve migraine headaches, though it's not clear exactly how they do this.

Six beta blockers have been found effective in preventing migraine headaches (see Table 2, page 20). The most effective medication varies from person to person, so if the first one doesn't work, it's worth trying another.

Side effects can include fatigue, dizziness, cold hands and feet, exercise intolerance, insomnia, shortness of breath, depression, and impotence. Some beta blockers can worsen asthma or other chronic lung disorders by narrowing the airways inside the lungs. They also may cause dangerously slow heart rates in unusual circumstances. Beta blockers may on occasion worsen heart failure, although they benefit most people with heart failure. People with heart and lung conditions who are on beta blockers should be closely monitored by a physician.

Tricyclics

Though typically used to treat depression, tricyclic medications (see Table 2, below) are sometimes prescribed for various types of pain, including headaches. Amitriptyline (Elavil, Endep) is the best studied for pain relief and the most often prescribed for migraine prevention: it's about 60% effective in thwarting such headaches. Other tricyclics used in migraine prevention include doxepin (Adapin, Sinequan), imipramine (Tofranil), and nortriptyline (Aventyl, Pamelor). It is not clear how these medications work, but it is possible that they relieve pain by increasing the availability of the neurotransmitters serotonin and norepinephrine, which not only affect mood but also act to reduce the transmission of pain signals in the brain.

When taking a tricyclic, you probably won't notice any benefit in the first week or two, and you may not feel its full effects for several weeks. However, some sedative effects are common early in treatment, which is a bonus for the many people with migraine who also have difficulty sleeping. Although a tricyclic could potentially improve mood, the doses prescribed for headache prevention are much lower than those used in treating depression. Side effects can include dry mouth, blurred vision, dizziness, weight gain, constipation, and difficulty urinating. People who have glaucoma, heart disease, or an enlarged prostate should not take these drugs.

Calcium-channel blockers

Like beta blockers, calcium-channel blockers (see Table 2, below) are often prescribed for people with

Table 2: Medications that help prevent migraine headaches

CLASS	GENERIC NAME (BRAND NAME)	SIDE EFFECTS	CAUTIONS
Beta blockers	atenolol (Tenormin) bisoprolol (Zebeta) metoprolol (Lopressor) nadolol (Corgard) propranolol (Inderal) timolol (Blocadren)	Fatigue, dizziness, depression, cold hands and feet, exercise intolerance, fatigue, insomnia, and impotence	People with heart failure, asthma, or other lung conditions should be closely monitored by a physician if they take these drugs. People taking thyroid medication should not take propranolol.
Tricyclic medications	amitriptyline (Elavil, Endep) doxepin (Adapin, Sinequan) imipramine (Tofranil) nortriptyline (Aventyl, Pamelor)	Drowsiness, dry mouth, blurred vision, weight gain, constipation, urinary retention	Do not take these drugs if you have glaucoma, heart disease, or an enlarged prostate, or if you are taking a monoamine oxidase inhibitor (MAOI) such as isocarboxazid (Marplan), phenelzine (Nardil), or tranylcypromine (Parnate).
Calcium-channel blockers	verapamil (Calan, Isoptin, Verelan)	Fatigue, dizziness, constipation, swollen ankles, and fluid retention	People with heart failure or problems with the electrical pathways in the heart should not take these drugs.
Anticonvulsants	divalproex (Depakote)	Nausea, diarrhea, weakness, tremor, and weight gain	People taking this medication need regular blood tests to monitor their liver function. Don't take this drug if you have any liver problems, including elevated liver enzyme levels.
	gabapentin (Neurontin)	Drowsiness, fatigue	Although this drug is not specifically approved for migraine headache treatment, doctors sometimes prescribe it to prevent migraine.
	topiramate (Topamax)	Drowsiness, loss of memory or thinking skills, weight loss, word-finding problems, tingling in hands and feet	Don't take this drug if you have a history of kidney stones.

high blood pressure or heart disease, as well as for migraine prevention. But these medications work in different ways. Calcium-channel blockers relax muscle cells in blood vessel walls and prevent blood vessel spasm, which is what first prompted scientists to investigate their value for migraine prevention. As it turns out, however, calcium-channel blockers prevent migraine not so much because they increase blood circulation, but because they act directly on nerve cells and thwart inflammation.

Treatment usually begins with a low dose of the most effective one, verapamil (Calan, others), that's increased gradually. Despite their name, calcium-channel blockers don't interfere with the absorption of calcium, nor do they cause calcium loss in the bones. Instead, they prevent the transmission of electrical signals—including pain signals—in the brain by blocking the calcium ion channels that must open before such signals pass from one cell to another. Side effects include fatigue, dizziness, constipation, and swelling of the feet. Calcium-channel blockers may not be the best choice for people with heart failure or heart rhythm abnormalities.

Anticonvulsants

The anticonvulsant, or antiseizure, medications topiramate (Topamax) and divalproex (Depakote) are among the few medications specifically approved for migraine prevention (see Table 2, page 20). Another anticonvulsant used for migraine prevention is gabapentin (Neurontin), even though it is not specifically FDA-approved for this use. Although the mechanisms are not entirely clear, anticonvulsants appear to work by reducing the transmission of pain signals in the brain.

Divalproex effectively prevents migraine headaches for about half of those who use it. However, beta blockers and tricyclic medications are generally more effective and better tolerated. Divalproex tends to be about as effective as calcium-channel blockers, although it's not as well tolerated. Its side effects can include nausea, diarrhea, weakness, weight gain, and tremor. Very rarely, it can cause potentially fatal liver failure. Consequently, people with liver disease shouldn't take this medication, and anyone who takes

divalproex should have regular liver function tests. Women who are pregnant or trying to become pregnant shouldn't take this drug.

Topiramate and gabapentin don't harm liver function, but these medications have other side effects to consider. One risk to keep in mind: topiramate may encourage the formation of kidney stones, so people taking it should drink plenty of fluids. Even so, topiramate and gabapentin offer an alternative for people who cannot tolerate or do not respond to divalproex. Studies show that topiramate reduces the frequency of migraine headaches, and these effects last at least six months, according to one report. Gabapentin has also proved effective for migraine prevention.

Aspirin

Results from the Physicians' Health Study suggest that aspirin also prevents migraines to some extent. The study, which involved 22,000 male physicians, found that men who took low-dose aspirin to reduce their risk of heart attacks also experienced roughly 20% fewer migraine headaches than those receiving a placebo.

Although low-dose aspirin is far less effective than the standard medicines for migraine prevention, it may improve migraine control when used in combination with one of the standard drugs, some researchers speculate. Because frequent aspirin use can irritate the stomach lining and cause internal bleeding, which can lead to anemia, consult your doctor before starting a daily aspirin regimen.

New approaches

What all of the medications above have in common is that they were developed for purposes other than migraine prevention. Now, however, drug companies are researching new therapies directed specifically at the underlying causes of migraine.

A class of so-called targeted therapies for migraine prevention has begun to show promise in the most rigorous type of studies: randomized, placebo-controlled clinical trials. Backed by more than three decades of research, these biological compounds target a chemical in the body called calcitonin gene-related peptide (CGRP) that's thought to play important roles in migraines. Research shows that CGRP, which is a compound that inflames nerve endings, is also one of the most potent vasodilators known. As blood vessels widen in response to CGRP, they press on nerves that trigger a pain response. And when activated, the nerves release more CGRP into the bloodstream. Studies show that blood levels of CGRP rise during migraine attacks and decline as a headache subsides.

CGRP-based therapies don't work fast enough to relieve a migraine that's already in progress. Instead, they're designed to prevent migraines by neutralizing CGRP for weeks at a time. The therapies are actually modified versions of natural compounds in the body. Called monoclonal antibodies, they work by binding to CGRP directly, thus blocking its activity, or by attaching to its receptor on nerve cells.

Four different CGRP-based therapies are in late-stage clinical trials and are nearing approval by the FDA for clinical use. These candidate therapies have demonstrated similar benefits in reducing headache frequency with few side effects. Some patients respond much more dramatically than the average, suggesting there may be "super-responders" to the effects of CGRP inhibition. Although the treatments are expected to be expensive, experts believe that CGRP-based therapies could help to fill a tremendous unmet medical need and revolutionize migraine prevention in much the same way that triptans revolutionized migraine treatment decades ago (see "Treating migraine pain," above right).

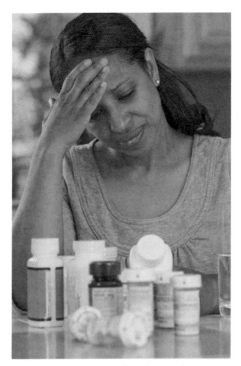

Steroids, antinausea medications, and magnetic devices are sometimes used for treating migraines. But the mainstay of treatment is a class of drugs known as triptans. They come in pill forms, injectables, and even a nasal spray.

© Huntstock | Thinkstock

Treating migraine pain

When prevention fails, a variety of self-help strategies (see page 25) can help get you through an attack, especially if the attacks are not frequent. But when migraines occur on a regular basis, it's time to speak with your doctor about a more powerful treatment.

Throughout history, migraine sufferers have endured an odd array of alleged remedies. Ancient Romans zapped headache pain with a jolt from a black torpedo fish, or electric ray. In the 13th century, Europeans tried opium as well as rub-on vinegar potions. In 1660, a gruesome procedure dating back to prehistoric times known as trepanation (drilling holes in the skull) was popularized as a migraine treatment by the English physician William Harvey. Even then, doctors understood that swelling blood vessels in the head played a role in migraine pain. Erasmus Darwin (grandfather of Charles Darwin) proposed yet another bizarre treatment: spinning the patient in a centrifuge to force the blood from the head to the feet.

Over the next two centuries, other theories about the origins of migraines arose, including the notion of migraine pain as a "nerve storm" within the brain, similar to epilepsy. Today, epilepsy drugs—the anticonvulsant medications mentioned earlier (see "Anticonvulsants," page 21)—are among those used to prevent migraines, though they aren't used for treating a migraine that's in progress.

The first drugs brought to market to treat migraine headaches, known as ergots, targeted the problem of dilated blood vessels, or vasodilation, with a substance based on rye fungus called ergotamine. During the 1940s, a semisynthetic version of ergotamine known as dihydroergotamine (DHE) came on the market and is still used today. Ergot-based drugs, such as Cafergot or Migranal, cause more side effects than newer medications, though, and are not commonly prescribed.

Ergots also take longer to work than newer drugs; however, their beneficial effect lasts longer, so users are less likely to suffer a headache recurrence. Ergotamine and caffeine suppositories or injectable DHE may be useful for severe headaches because they're absorbed faster than ergots in traditional pill form, and a nasal spray version of DHE (Migranal Nasal Spray) is also available but much less effective.

Fortunately for migraine sufferers, newer, better drugs and delivery systems are available today.

Triptans: Migraine mainstays

Drug developers created triptan drugs in an effort to make a medication that worked similarly to ergots but caused fewer side effects. Like ergots, the triptans work by constricting dilated blood vessels. In addition, they block the release of chemicals that inflame the dilated blood vessels. By 1991, the first of these drugs, sumatriptan (Imitrex), was approved by the FDA. First available only by injection, triptans are now available as pills, melt-in-the-mouth tablets, nasal sprays, skin patches, and needle-free injectables as well. A total of seven triptans and one combination product with a triptan are on the market today, including a variety of second-generation products designed for faster, more efficient absorption and better tolerability (see Table 3, below). Triptans relieve pain far faster than ergots, with improvements start-ing in 20 to 30 minutes and complete relief within one to two hours.

In pill form, almotriptan (Axert), eletriptan (Relpax), rizatriptan (Maxalt), sumatriptan (Imitrex), or zolmitriptan (Zomig) can stop a migraine within two hours, provided the drug is taken when the headache is still mild. Doctors stress the importance of taking the drug as soon as possible after your symptoms begin, because as a migraine headache progresses, it slows down the function of the gastrointestinal system so the medications aren't absorbed as well (see Figure 7, page 24). Although naratriptan (Amerge) and frovatriptan (Frova) can take nearly twice as long to work, they have fewer side effects and are more effective in preventing a migraine's return within 24 hours.

Several alternative delivery systems have been developed for triptans. These include an automatic injectable form of sumatriptan (Imitrex Statdose, Zembrace, Alsuma) that can provide relief in as little as 15 minutes and may be self-administered. A needle-free system of sumatriptan (Sumavel DosePro) is available that delivers a fine burst of compressed nitrogen to push the drug through the skin into the bloodstream. It is as effective and fast-acting as the injectable form, but while it avoids needles, it is more likely to cause minor swelling, bruising, redness, and bleeding.

Sumatriptan and zolmitriptan also come in nasal sprays (Imitrex Nasal Spray, Zomig Nasal Spray) that are absorbed within an hour, making them a good choice for more intense migraine headaches. However, one problem with nasal sprays is that much of the medication ends up being swallowed instead of absorbed through the nasal lining. A unique breath-powered delivery system for sumatriptan (Onzetra Xsail), approved in 2016, helps solve that problem. You blow into one end of the device, propelling a fast-acting powder form of the medication out the other end, inserted in your nostril. The powder goes up your nose, where it is rapidly absorbed. Furthermore, the act of blowing closes the epiglottis and prevents the medication from being swallowed.

It's not unusual to experience some mild side effects when taking triptans. The oral medications can cause a tingling in your fingers or tightness in your

Table 3: Triptans

GENERIC NAME (BRAND NAME)	SIDE EFFECTS	CAUTIONS AND COMMENTS
almotriptan (Axert)	Tingling in the fingers or tightness in the throat, muscle tightness, burning or soreness in the nose (nasal spray), dizziness, dry mouth, muscle aches, cramps, nausea, vomiting	People with heart disease or uncontrolled high blood pressure should not take these medications.
eletriptan (Relpax)		
frovatriptan (Frova)		
naratriptan (Amerge)		
rizatriptan (Maxalt)		
sumatriptan (Imitrex, Sumavel DosePro, Zecuity)		
sumatriptan and naproxen sodium (Treximet)		
zolmitriptan (Zomig)		

Figure 7: Why migraine headaches make you nauseated

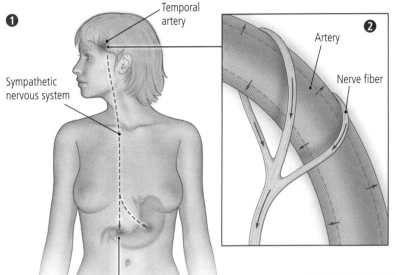

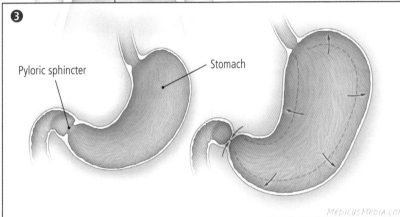

❶ During a migraine headache, arteries in the head (especially in the temporal area) dilate.

❷ The widened arteries stretch nerve fibers that encircle the arteries, causing them to send impulses to the brain. In turn, these nerve impulses cause pain and activate the sympathetic nervous system (SNS), which originates in the spinal cord and extends to organs throughout the body, including the stomach and intestines. The SNS controls the body's "fight or flight" response, mobilizing the body for action by speeding up the heart rate, raising blood pressure, and slowing digestion.

❸ To slow digestion, the SNS closes the pyloric sphincter (the ring of smooth muscle that separates the stomach from the upper part of the intestines). As a result, the stomach dilates and any leftover food stays in the stomach, which can cause the nausea and vomiting that often accompany migraine headaches. This phenomenon also explains why migraine medications taken by mouth aren't very effective—this slowdown delays their absorption into the bloodstream.

throat, while the nasal spray can leave a bad taste in your mouth. The injectable form of sumatriptan tends to cause more intense side effects, and also tends to cause muscle tightness, which can temporarily worsen the headache or cause chest pressure.

If one triptan doesn't work, another often will (although you may have to wait 24 hours before taking a different type). If your headache still isn't completely relieved, taking aspirin or another NSAID—such as ibuprofen, naproxen, or ketoprofen (see "Over-the-counter pain relievers," page 28)—along with the triptan may help. Another option is a drug that combines sumatriptan and naproxen sodium (Treximet), which was approved for migraines with or without auras in 2008. Studies showed that more people who took Treximet for migraine pain experienced relief than

those who took either sumatriptan or naproxen alone.

From 30% to 40% of the time, the headache returns within 24 hours of taking a triptan medication. Depending on the dose, you may be able to take the same triptan again during a given 24-hour period, but you can't take another triptan, too, or a similarly working ergot. Because triptans and ergots temporarily narrow blood vessels, taking them at the same time could lead to a heart attack. Not surprisingly, people with heart disease or uncontrolled high blood pressure shouldn't take these medications.

Other options

For people who can't take triptans because of side effects or other potential problems, several other types of medications may help. These medications are not as commonly used for migraines, however, and should be used with caution. Magnetic devices may also help. There are also various low-tech, self-help techniques to try during a migraine attack (see "Self-help strategies for migraine sufferers," below).

Steroids. Occasionally, a migraine headache is exceptionally stubborn: despite treatment, it may persist for days or weeks. When this happens, a several-day course of a steroid, such as prednisone, may provide relief.

Antinausea medications. Migraine attacks often activate the sympathetic nervous system, which is probably best known for its role in the "fight or flight" response. Activating the sympathetic nervous system affects the stomach as well as other parts of the body (see Figure 7, page 24). As a result, migraine headaches often provoke nausea, and in some cases vomiting, which can prevent you from keeping down your medications. Even when vomiting does not occur, the stomach takes longer to empty into the intestines once the sympathetic nervous system is activated—which can impair the absorption of oral medications.

To prevent vomiting, your doctor may recommend a prescription antinausea medication. Several options exist. The phenothiazines suppress nausea and—because they have sedative effects—also help you sleep. The antinausea medication metoclopramide (Reglan) helps empty the stomach, thereby improving the absorption of oral headache medications. Many people find it particularly effective to take metoclopramide at the first hint of a migraine headache and then, about 15 minutes later, to take the first dose of headache medication. Virtually all the antinausea drugs are available in several forms. If you can't take them by mouth, you can try rectal suppositories and, in extreme cases, injections.

Prescription painkillers. Prescription painkillers are more powerful than their over-the-counter

equivalents, yet they rarely relieve severe migraine pain. In many cases, prescription formulations just provide higher doses of standard nonprescription products, such as ibuprofen or naproxen sodium. Some prescription painkillers contain barbiturates or opioids. Opioids, such as codeine and morphine, are generally avoided in the treatment of headaches. People who regularly use opioids run the risk of developing "rebound" headaches when the medication is stopped. They may also develop a tolerance to the drugs, meaning they need higher and higher doses to relieve the pain. In addition, they may become dependent, meaning they develop withdrawal symptoms when they stop taking the medication.

In rare instances, people will progress to opioid addiction, which compels them to do whatever they can to obtain the drugs, no matter what consequences they may suffer. Barbiturates, a class of sedatives that contain butalbital, are also controversial as migraine treatments because they, too, are prone to abuse; however, they can help some people when other treatments fail.

Magnetic devices. One way to relieve a migraine headache without medication is with a technique called transcranial magnetic stimulation (TMS). This treatment delivers magnetic pulses through the back

Self-help strategies for migraine sufferers

To help ease symptoms, try these home remedies:

- Lie down, preferably in a dark, quiet room.
- Place a cold compress (an ice pack, bag of ice cubes, or bag of frozen vegetables, wrapped in a towel) on your head and a heating pad or warm towel on the back of the neck and shoulders.
- Sip ginger ale to ease nausea and replace any fluids lost from vomiting.
- If your headache is especially bad, take a medication that makes you drowsy—a sleeping pill or the nonprescription allergy drug diphenhydramine (Benadryl).

For additional ideas, see the Special Section, "Self-help and alternative strategies to ease headache pain," page 27.

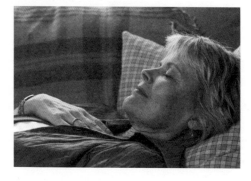

of the skull directly into a part of the brain called the occipital cortex, where a migraine starts, before it creeps toward other parts of the brain involved in sensation and hearing.

A TMS device called SpringTMS has been approved by the FDA for both preventing migraines and treating migraines with an aura. The device requires a prescription, but it's easy and painless to use: you simply hold it with both hands against your head, and release magnetic pulses by pressing a button.

In a clinical study of 201 people, nearly 34% of those who used the device to relieve a migraine were pain-free, even after 24 hours, compared with about 10% of control subjects who used a sham device that didn't emit the magnetic signal. The device didn't relieve other migraine symptoms, such as nausea or sensitivity to light and sound. And it also had occasional side effects, including vertigo (dizziness). You should never use the device if you have metal in your head, neck, or upper body, or if you have a pacemaker, all of which can be pulled out of place with the magnet. Similarly, you shouldn't use it if you've been diagnosed with epilepsy or have a family history of seizures. ♥

Self-help and alternative strategies to ease headache pain

Whether headaches are an occasional annoyance or a frequent ailment for you, a range of remedies and self-help strategies may help to ease them. Some are things you can do on your own—for example, avoiding the foods, activities, or situations that trigger your headaches; using mind-body techniques such as yoga or meditation to reduce your stress; or trying herbal supplements (see Table 4, page 29). Even something as simple as a cup of coffee may help. Other approaches, like acupuncture or physical therapy, require you to seek out a specialist.

These strategies are not always substitutes for prescription treatments. But even if these techniques don't provide complete relief, they can complement other medical care and may enable you to cut back on medications. Check with your health insurance plan before trying any therapies that cost you money, because some may not be covered. You may also want to discuss them with your doctor to help find the treatments that best fit your needs.

Aspirin and other pain relievers

When most people get a headache, they reach for whatever painkiller they happen to have in their medicine cabinet. And most of the time, an over-the-counter (OTC) pain reliever will do the trick (see "Over-the-counter pain relievers," page 28). This easy, effective strategy is fine for people who have mild to moderately painful headaches once in a while. But if you need to take an OTC painkiller more than a

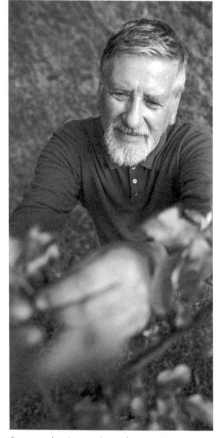

Stress reduction and regular exercise can both help reduce the frequency and severity of headaches. Gardening is one particularly pleasant way to get some of both.

couple of times a week, that means you're suffering from regular, rather than occasional, headaches, and you should see your doctor. Also, talk to your doctor if OTC medications fail to ease your pain.

© ViktorCap | Thinkstock

These drugs are not strong enough for many people with severe headaches; however, a prescription drug may provide relief, as described elsewhere in this report.

Avoiding triggers

This technique is simple, poses no risks, and costs nothing. The first step is to figure out whether there's a connection between your headaches and particular foods, activities, or situations. Few triggers are obvious, so a headache diary is a good tool to use when trying to identify yours (see "Keeping a headache diary," page 8). For common triggers of migraines, see "Common triggers," page 18, and "Migraines and food," page 19.

If you do find that certain foods, beverages, smells, activities, or other things bring on your headaches, make it a priority to avoid these triggers. For example, people with cluster headaches usually find that they need to give up alcohol during periods when their headaches are active. Wearing blue- or green-tinted sunglasses can help fend off an attack if your headaches are triggered by sunlight. Or if changes in eating and sleeping habits are likely to set off a headache, make an extra effort to stick to a regular schedule.

Even after you identify triggers, the amount of control you'll have over your headaches will vary. Avoiding triggers isn't always easy. For example, chocolate and the food additive monosodium glutamate (MSG) trigger headaches in some people, but many processed foods contain MSG, and it can be difficult to give up a favorite treat such as chocolate. On the other hand, you may be able to lessen headache frequency without eliminating certain triggers altogether, or you may find that triggers interact with one another in ways that make them more manageable. For instance, you may find that chocolate or alcohol provokes a headache only if you haven't had enough rest or if you consume it on an empty stomach.

Exercise

Regular exercise helps keep the heart and blood vessels healthy. It also boosts your mood, relieves stress, and helps prevent a host of ailments, such as diabetes and high

---

Over-the-counter pain relievers

Many headache formulas found in drugstores fall into one of the three categories below; others combine these drugs with other substances. Excedrin, for instance, includes acetaminophen, aspirin, and caffeine.

Regardless of which medication you choose, follow the directions carefully. Taking too much medication, even over-the-counter pain relievers, can actually make your headaches worse. There are a couple reasons for this. The pills only address the pain, allowing the underlying mechanisms to worsen over time. In addition, continual use of these remedies can cause your body's natural pain-quenching system to become lazy. Over time, you'll need stronger doses of medication to get relief—and when the medicine wears off, you may develop a "rebound" headache (see "Medication overuse headaches," page 33).

Acetaminophen. Acetaminophen (Tylenol and others) is a generally safe non-aspirin pain reliever. But beware that doses above 3 grams (3,000 mg) per day, especially when combined with alcohol, can cause potentially fatal liver damage. If you consume three or more alcoholic drinks a day, every day, don't take acetaminophen.

Aspirin. Aspirin quells pain and may prevent migraine headaches in some people when taken regularly. Long-term side effects include kidney damage and gastrointestinal problems, such as stomach pain, heartburn, or nausea. Bleeding from the stomach can also occur, often in such minute quantities as to go unnoticed. However, over time anemia may result, causing fatigue—which, in turn, may increase the frequency of headaches. Avoid aspirin if you have reflux, gastritis, or ulcers. Aspirin belongs to a group of drugs called nonsteroidal anti-inflammatory drugs (NSAIDs).

Other NSAIDs. Besides aspirin, NSAIDs include ibuprofen (Advil, Motrin, others), naproxen sodium (Aleve, Anaprox), and ketoprofen (Actron, Orudis, others), but not acetaminophen. In some people, these drugs help prevent migraine headaches. In 2015, the FDA warned that unlike aspirin, they can raise the risk of heart attacks and strokes, particularly with prolonged use. People with heart disease should avoid taking them, and others should try to limit the dose and duration of use; long-term users should consider taking "holidays" from the drugs.

Table 4: Herbal and other dietary supplements for headache pain

The following are some of the most widely used preparations for headaches. Note that the FDA does not regulate the effectiveness or safety of these products. Consult your doctor before taking any of these supplements, as they can interact with medications to treat headaches or other conditions.

NAME	WHAT IT IS	EVIDENCE FOR USE	SIDE EFFECTS AND CAUTIONS
Feverfew	A daisy-like flower native to Europe. The dried leaves (and sometimes flowers and stems) are used to make capsules, tablets, and extracts.	Limited evidence suggests that 50 to 100 mg daily of feverfew extract can reduce the frequency of migraine headaches.	May cause mouth inflammation or ulceration. Feverfew can enhance the effect of medications that cause bleeding, such as aspirin and warfarin (Coumadin). Do not take if you have a history of heart disease, bleeding disorders, or anxiety.
Magnesium	A mineral found in legumes, whole grains, vegetables (especially broccoli, squash, and green leafy vegetables), seeds, and nuts (especially almonds); also available as a supplement. For adults ages 30 and older, the Recommended Dietary Allowance (RDA) is 420 mg for men and 320 mg for women.	People with cluster headaches or migraines (especially menstrual migraines) tend to have low magnesium levels. One study found that a 600-mg daily supplement helped reduce migraine frequency.	Mild gastrointestinal effects, especially diarrhea. Do not take if you have kidney problems.
Vitamin B_2 (riboflavin)	A vitamin found mainly in milk and other dairy products and whole and enriched grains and cereals; also available in supplement form. The RDA for men is 1.3 mg; for women, 1.1 mg.	Very high daily doses (400 mg) of riboflavin reduced migraine frequency in one three-month study.	Diarrhea and frequent urination.
Coenzyme Q_{10} (CoQ$_{10}$)	A vitamin-like substance found in small amounts in all human cells, as well as in small amounts in a variety of foods.	Limited evidence suggests that 150 to 300 mg of CoQ$_{10}$ daily lessens migraine frequency.	Possible nausea. May lower blood pressure. Use with caution if you have diabetes or a bleeding disorder.
Peppermint oil	A popular culinary herb; extracts and oil from the stems, leaves, and flowers are also used to flavor toothpaste and many other products.	Rubbing small amounts of peppermint oil into the temples may help relieve the symptoms of tension headaches.	Keep the oil away from your eyes, and watch for allergic reactions; use caution if you have sensitive skin or asthma.

blood pressure. Virtually any type of physical activity, if performed regularly, can help prevent headaches.

For overall health benefits, most experts recommend 30 minutes of moderate activity—such as brisk walking, yoga, gardening, or bike riding—every day or nearly every day. It's important to note, though, that strenuous physical activity, such as running (especially in hot, humid weather), can provoke migraine headaches in susceptible people.

Psychotherapy

Scientists once associated headaches with particular personality types or underlying psychological problems, but research has largely discounted such notions. Nonetheless, a type of psychotherapy called cognitive behavioral therapy (CBT) can sometimes ease headaches or help you cope with them. CBT is a directed form of psychotherapy that focuses on practical strategies and habits to bring about behavioral change—in this case, to manage headaches and to forestall or cope with the effects of headache pain on your life. CBT can be particularly helpful for people whose headaches are exacerbated by stress, anxiety, or depression. The negative thoughts about headaches and how they affect your life can take a toll, interfering with daily activities or causing worry and stress that worsen the problem. CBT helps you identify and change negative thought patterns.

Other types of psychotherapy may help, too. Depression and headaches are frequent companions. A psychological evaluation can sometimes identify depression that's obscured by pain or that produces subtle symptoms. In such circumstances, an antidepressant may help. People who suffer from both depression and headaches may respond better to a combination of psychotherapy and medication than to medication alone, even if the headaches improve significantly with just the medication.

Mind-body techniques

Mind-body therapies—such as meditation, relaxation techniques, yoga, hypnosis, stress management, and biofeedback—seek to harness the power of the mind to aid in health and pain relief. These techniques are quite popular with Americans suffering from headaches: half use some type of mind-body technique to alleviate the pain, and many of them find it very helpful.

Which techniques will be most useful for you? That may depend on your personal preferences, as well as the type of headaches you have. Two techniques that have been used for headache treatment are relaxation training and biofeedback, which can be used alone or in combination with CBT. A 2017 review found a noticeable benefit from mind-body therapies—particularly relaxation training combined with CBT—for people with chronic migraines.

Stress is a widely accepted trigger of headaches, which may occur during periods of stress or just after a stressful event. Mind-body techniques lower stress, and they also promote healthier lifestyle habits, such as getting adequate sleep, which can help to keep headaches at bay. Still, questions remain about which specific approaches work best for headache sufferers—and how often and how long to pursue them.

Relaxation techniques

A number of techniques can relax your muscles and ease tension, which should help reduce headache pain. No single relaxation technique works better than the others, so it's best to experiment until you find the approach that helps you the most. Whichever technique you choose, it will work only if you do it on a regular basis, preferably daily. Options include these:

- **Deep diaphragmatic breathing:** slow, controlled breathing in which your abdomen (rather than your chest) expands with each breath. This technique is most relaxing if you make the exhalation longer than the inhalation.

- **Meditation:** a process of sitting quietly and directing your attention to a single point of focus, such as the breath, a phrase, or bodily sensations. Small studies have found that a structured meditation-based program called Mindfulness-Based Stress Reduction, which cultivates an awareness of the present moment, can help reduce pain and improve quality of life in migraine sufferers.

- **Visualization:** a practice in which you imagine a peaceful scene that relaxes you. Some people find this easier to do with a recording, video, or counselor who guides you through the practice.

- **Hypnotherapy:** a relaxation technique performed by a therapist that has been shown in a handful of studies to help reduce the frequency of migraines in both children and adults. Hypnosis is not a form of sleep but a state of deep relaxation, during which the therapist suggests visualizations that help ease pain. To find a qualified hypnotherapist, seek one who is licensed in your state and is a member of the American Society of Clinical Hypnosis or the Society for Clinical and

A prescription for stress relief

You can't eliminate stress from your life, but a few tried-and-true coping techniques may help prevent headaches or ease them once they begin.

- **Exercise.** Aerobic exercise alleviates stress and can boost your mood. Aim to work 30 minutes of moderate activity, such as brisk walking, into your schedule on all or most days.

- **Get enough sleep.** Most people need seven to eight hours of sleep a night. If you're finding it hard to fall or stay asleep, you may want to examine your waking hours. Strategies such as exercising early in the day, avoiding caffeine in the afternoon, limiting fluids before bedtime, and not watching TV in bed can improve sleep. If you still have trouble sleeping, consider consulting a sleep specialist.

- **Learn relaxation techniques.** Try meditation, yoga, or deep breathing.

- **Confront stressful situations head-on.** Don't wait until the end of the day or week to confront a problem. Use negotiation skills at work, and hold family problem-solving sessions at home.

- **Improve your time-management skills.** These techniques can help you juggle work and family demands and ease your stress levels.

- **Treat yourself to a massage every so often.** Research shows that massage can lead to pain relief and a better state of mind, especially among people who suffer from chronic tension headaches.

Experimental Hypnosis (see "Resources," page 38). These are the only nationally recognized organizations for licensed health care professionals using hypnosis.

Biofeedback

Biofeedback involves using a machine to monitor body functioning, as indicated by finger temperature or electrical activity in muscles. The machine then translates the readings into a blinking light, a beeping sound, or a graph. People can gauge how their bodies are reacting by observing these signals. They are then taught relaxation exercises and thought patterns to change and control those reactions. The goal is to be able to consciously control a particular body function and hence relax.

Two types of biofeedback are commonly used to manage headaches:

- surface electromyography, which measures electrical activity in a muscle via electrodes placed on the skin
- thermal biofeedback, which measures finger temperature.

Biofeedback should be undertaken only with the help of a skilled professional. It's not wise to pick someone based on a Web search or to buy biofeedback equipment found through an advertisement or a mail-order catalog. Instead, ask your doctor for a referral. Biofeedback works best as an element of a treatment plan that also includes medication.

Acupuncture

According to traditional Chinese beliefs, acupuncture works by affecting the flow of energy, called *qi*, through pathways that run through the body. The practitioner inserts very fine needles at specific points along these pathways, which are known as meridians. Although acupuncture has many variations, it typically involves four to 10 needles that are left in place for 10 to 30 minutes, while you lie in a darkened room. A course of treatment may include six to 12 sessions. Most people report that acupuncture needles cause little or no pain.

Acupuncture has long been used to manage headaches, but recent evidence lends scientific support to this application of an ancient practice. A 2016 review from the Cochrane Collaboration (an international organization that provides comprehensive reviews of medical literature) concluded that acupuncture is at least as effective as medication for preventing migraine attacks. The review examined studies involving people who received either real acupuncture or a sham procedure in which needles were either inserted at incorrect points or didn't penetrate the skin. Overall, participants in these studies experienced relief from both approaches, but the real acupuncture had a small additional benefit over the sham treatment. When acupuncture was compared with drug treatments, the acupuncture reduced headache frequency slightly more, but the difference was less pronounced over time. People who received acupuncture reported fewer adverse effects.

A separate Cochrane review of studies on the use of acupuncture for preventing tension headaches, also published in 2016, found a similar beneficial effect, with about half of patients experiencing at least a 50% reduction in headache frequency with acupuncture, slightly more than a sham treatment. Further studies are needed to compare acupuncture against other treatments for tension headaches.

While correct needle placement seems less relevant than most acupuncturists believe, the treatment appears to be among the most promising of nontraditional headache therapies.

If you'd like to try acupuncture, do your homework before choosing a practitioner. Licensing requirements vary from state to state. If possible, choose a therapist with a state license. All needles should be disposable or properly sterilized before use. If you live in a state that doesn't require licensing, seek out a practitioner who's certified by the National Certification Commis-

sion for Acupuncture and Oriental Medicine (see "Resources," page 38). You may also want to get a referral from your doctor, as some insurance companies will cover acupuncture for migraines.

Physical therapy, massage, chiropractic, osteopathy

By relaxing the tense muscles that commonly accompany tension and migraine headaches, certain types of physical interventions may provide relief, including physical therapy, massage, chiropractic treatments, and osteopathic manipulation treatment.

A physical therapist can evaluate your posture to see if a problem with your neck positioning needs to be corrected, and can teach you daily neck and shoulder exercises you can do on your own. In addition, he or she will likely use one or more office-based treatments, such as the following:

- ultrasound, which uses a device that emits sound waves that penetrate the skin and warm muscle tissue
- electrical nerve stimulation, which employs a battery-powered device to send electrical signals to underlying nerves
- traction, which involves using a special device to stretch a tight muscle, usually in the neck
- myofascial release, which involves performing a series of massage-like techniques to stretch tight muscles.

Physical therapists often use hot or cold compresses as well. You can try the same techniques at home. To prevent headaches, for example, a heating pad applied daily to the back of the neck or shoulders can relax tense muscles. Taking a hot shower or bath can also help but does not work as well as using a heating pad daily.

For a headache already in progress, cold is better. A cold pack can constrict blood vessels and can be especially helpful for throbbing temples.

Massage, when performed by a licensed massage therapist, can also loosen tight muscles. However, be aware that certain techniques can worsen headaches. For instance, although gentle massage can provide headache relief for some people, a too-firm or aggressive massage can actually bring on a severe headache.

Chiropractic treatment is also sometimes used to relieve migraines and headaches resulting from problems in the cervical spine (the upper part of the spine, in the neck area).

Osteopathy, with its more gentle manipulations, may also ease pain, according to a systematic review published in 2017. But more research is needed to determine its effectiveness. Osteopathy is performed by a doctor of osteopathic medicine (D.O.), who is trained in both conventional medicine and osteopathic techniques. ▼

Chronic headaches

Although most people experience headaches from time to time, an unfortunate but significant minority—about one in 20 people—experience them daily or almost daily for a prolonged period of time. Having headaches at least 15 days a month for a year or longer is a condition called chronic headache.

In two out of three cases, chronic headaches develop in people who have experienced only intermittent migraine, tension, or other types of headaches. Then over the course of a decade or so, their headaches gradually increase in frequency until they occur on a near-daily basis. In the remaining one-third of cases, chronic headaches develop without warning—sometimes as a result of illness, surgery, or an injury to the head, neck, or back, and sometimes for no apparent reason. Women are twice as likely as men to develop this severely debilitating disorder.

Regardless of the cause, chronic headaches are notoriously difficult to treat and, understandably, often produce anxiety and depression. To make matters worse, about half of people with chronic headaches have chronic migraines, which are intensely painful. The other half have chronic tension headaches, which tend to be less severe. In virtually all cases, people with chronic migraines (but not necessarily chronic tension headaches) have additional health problems, such as fibromyalgia, irritable bowel syndrome, or restless legs syndrome. It's actually unusual for doctors to diagnose or treat chronic migraines in people who have no additional health problems. These other conditions should also be addressed during treatment, along with any anxiety or depression.

The types of headaches you've had in the past may affect your symptoms. Migraine sufferers who develop chronic migraines may find that the pain starts to resemble the steady, vise-like grip of tension headaches. In addition, the aura often diminishes, although the throbbing at the temples that's typical

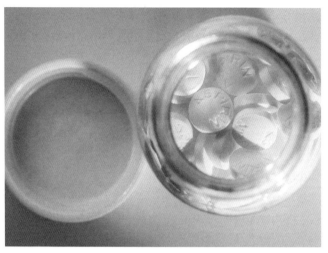

Ironically, overuse of pain relievers can contribute to chronic headaches. The problem is often caffeine-containing drugs that lead to a type of rebound headache when the caffeine wears off.

of migraines frequently continues. Meanwhile, those with a history of tension headaches often develop nausea and vomiting, sensitivity to light and noise, and throbbing in the temples—all hallmarks of migraines.

Medication overuse headaches

As many as 50% to 80% of chronic headache sufferers say they use pain relievers frequently—which, paradoxically, may make their headaches worse over time and can drive them to become daily occurrences.

This common headache type, known as medication overuse headache, can occur with excessive use of any headache medication, but caffeine-containing drugs are most often to blame (see Table 5, page 34). Contrary to popular belief, caffeine has a long-lasting effect and can stay in your system for two to three days, although this varies from person to person. If you take caffeine-containing medications more than two to three times a week, it is thought that the vasoconstricting effect (making your blood vessels constrict, or tighten) may build up. Then, when the caffeine wears off, your blood vessels expand again, reigniting

© Warrenrandalcarr | Thinkstock

your headache—an effect similar to a "weekend headache" (see "Unusual headaches," page 3). The phenomenon, also known as a drug rebound headache, is less common with triptan drugs because they don't stay in your system as long—usually only 12 hours or so.

In addition to the rebound vasodilation (expansion of blood vessels), experts also speculate that the regular use of pain relievers interferes with the body's natural painkilling system. Because pain medications mask symptoms, whatever is causing the pain may worsen. As the pain becomes more intense, pain relievers have less ability to control it, which can cause a great deal of frustration. But aside from worsening the pain, medication overuse headaches are not thought to be dangerous, and only rarely does medication overuse turn into a drug dependency.

People with medication-induced chronic headaches may experience severe pain upon awakening, which then lessens as the day goes on—the reverse of the pattern most often seen in chronic headaches.

Such severe morning headaches probably result because any medication taken during the day has worn off during the night. The pain then subsides during the day as additional medication is taken.

Managing chronic headaches

Treatment for chronic headaches aims to reduce their frequency so that they become intermittent and, at the same time, to alleviate the disruption and disability the headaches cause.

As part of that management strategy, your health care provider may recommend a daily medication for headache prevention. Such drugs are thought to work by altering brain chemistry to make you less susceptible. The options include medications that are "borrowed" from other disease categories—including blood pressure drugs (see "Beta blockers," page 19, and "Calcium-channel blockers," page 20), seizure drugs (see "Anticonvulsants," page 21), antidepressants (see Tricyclics," page 20), and others that have also been found to help people with chronic headaches.

Sometimes a drug combination works better than a single medication. One effective strategy is to combine a tricyclic medication with a beta blocker. This approach helps prevent both daily tension headaches and frequent migraine headaches, because the beta blocker decreases the intensity of headaches, while the tricyclic reduces their frequency. For both tension and migraine headaches, some doctors may also recommend a short-acting muscle relaxant, or a longer-acting muscle relaxant taken before bed. If you have trouble sleeping at night, ask your doctor whether you might take a tricyclic such as amitriptyline (Elavil, Endep) or doxepin (Adapin, Sinequan), which can induce drowsiness, thereby helping both headache and sleep problems. If sleeping difficulties are not an issue, imipramine (Tofranil) or nortriptyline (Pamelor) are other options. Any of the beta blockers listed in Table 2 (page 20) can be used in combination with a tricyclic medication.

You may also be prescribed a triptan or other medication that's designed to stop headaches when they do strike, sometimes called an abortive treatment. The preventive medication may help reduce

Table 5: Caffeine content of some common headache drugs

Caffeine is a double-edged sword when it comes to headache drugs. While this popular stimulant helps pain relievers work more quickly and efficiently, it is often a suspect in medication overuse headaches. (Note: For comparison's sake, the caffeine content in a cup of coffee ranges from 95 to 200 milligrams.)

DRUG NAME	CAFFEINE CONTENT (MG)
Over-the-counter drugs	
Anacin Advanced Headache Formula	65
Excedrin Migraine	65
Goody's Extra Strength Headache Powders	32.5
Midol Complete Caplets	60
Vanquish Extra-Strength Pain Reliever Caplets	33
Prescription drugs	
Fioricet (acetaminophen, butalbital, caffeine)	40
Fiorinal (aspirin, butalbital, caffeine)	40
Norgesic (aspirin, caffeine, orphenadrine)	30
Norgesic Forte (aspirin, caffeine, orphenadrine)	60
Synalgos-DC (aspirin, caffeine, dihydrocodeine)	30

Botulinum toxin for chronic migraines

Botulinum toxin (Botox, Dysport, Xeomin, others) is well known as a wrinkle-buster; injecting tiny amounts above the eyes and over the bridge of the nose relaxes small areas of muscles, smoothing crow's feet and frown lines. The effect is caused by a toxin produced by the bacterium *Clostridium botulinum*, which binds to nerve endings. Before it became a cosmetic treatment, the toxin was more commonly associated with botulism, a rare but serious paralytic illness that can afflict people who eat food contaminated with the toxin. In spite of its potent toxicity, botulinum toxin has been safely used and approved for a variety of medical applications, including the treatment of cross-eye, abnormal squinting and eyelid twitching, neck and shoulder muscle spasms, and severe sweating.

In the mid-1990s, a number of anecdotal reports suggested that people who got botulinum toxin injections to reduce wrinkles had fewer migraine headaches, spurring a flurry of clinical trials to test that idea. The conclusion so far is that it is "probably ineffective" as a treatment for occasional migraines and chronic tension headaches—but potentially useful for chronic migraines, for which the FDA has approved the use of Botox (but not other botulinum toxin products). However, the effect of the treatment is small, lowering the number of days sufferers have migraines by only about 15%.

If you are a potential candidate for this therapy, be sure to find a physician with experience doing the injections. Doctors require extensive training to properly administer the required 31 injections in seven different areas of the head and neck.

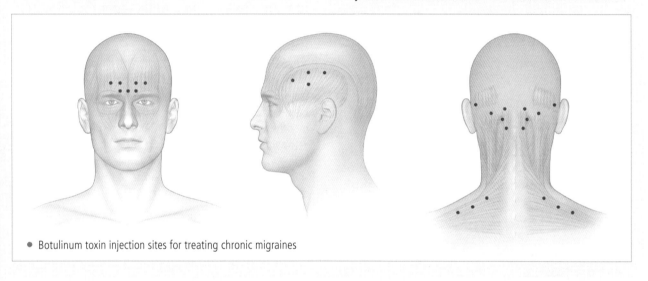

● Botulinum toxin injection sites for treating chronic migraines

headache frequency so you need an abortive treatment less often.

Abortive medications are not meant to be used daily. Depending on the particular drug, taking more than 10 to 15 doses in a month for several months may set you up for medication overuse headaches. If your headaches begin to get worse rather than better when you use abortive treatments, talk to your doctor. It may be best to stop the overused medication and start over with more appropriate headache management, including a preventive drug or drug combination that's safer to take every day. Your doctor can say whether it's best to quit the abortive medication abruptly or taper off slowly. You may experience side effects during the withdrawal process, such as nausea, vomiting, and muscle pain in the neck and shoulder

areas. If side effects are severe, your doctor can prescribe medications to alleviate them during the withdrawal period.

If you suffer from chronic migraines, then your doctor should also treat any additional health problems that might be triggering your headaches or making them worse, such as anxiety, depression, insomnia, or physical ailments such as irritable bowel syndrome or restless legs syndrome. These additional ailments (known medically as comorbidities) interact with headaches in complicated ways. For instance, evidence shows that anxiety can trigger migraines, which in turn can lead to depression. Similarly, chronic migraines can lead to insomnia, which itself is a risk factor for chronic migraines. Treatments for insomnia, such as cognitive behavioral therapy (see "Psychotherapy," page 29), may

Coping with chronic migraines: One woman's story

Monique Albert (not her real name), 47, used to work as a commercial pilot for a major airline while suffering with migraines, though they had not yet been diagnosed. She lives on Cape Cod. Following is her story.

In my preteens, I was the kid who had a lot of headaches, but I would take a Tylenol or Excedrin and the headache would go away. It was pretty much like that until my mid-30s. By then I had two children, and maybe it was hormonal or just the stress of having kids, but it all started getting worse.

Though I didn't know it yet, I was having migraines. My headaches are mostly on the left side. Sometimes the pain is right around my temple, and sometimes it feels like a tight headband around my head. Sometimes I get discomfort along the left side of my nose, or right behind my left eye, which is the worst of all. I'm definitely a high-stress person, and if I'm in a situation that's stressful, boom, I have a headache. Smells really trigger my headaches. I can't be around perfume or strong-smelling hairspray or fresh paint or diesel smells.

During a flight 10 years ago, I had a sudden pain on the left side of my head. It got so severe we actually ended up diverting the airplane. I went to the ER and they did a CT scan and saw a little sinus congestion. They thought it was a sinus infection and sent me home with an antibiotic, and that was the end of the episode. Fortunately, I've never experienced anything like that again.

After that incident, I went on medical leave to figure out what was going on. At one point I had literally 10 different specialists. I went to the dentist for TMJ disorder and got a mouth guard because I was clenching my teeth at night. My primary care doctor sent me to an infectious disease specialist, and I tested positive for Lyme disease and got treated with an antibiotic. I got the clearance to go back to work. However, none of these treatments cured my headaches.

Then in 2009, I got furloughed from the airline, and I had the time again to start searching again for an answer. I ended up at the headache clinic at Brigham and Women's Faulkner Hospital in Boston, where I was diagnosed with chronic migraine headaches. It was a relief to have a name for the discomfort I've been experiencing for a good part of my life.

Over the years, I've been on a zillion different prescriptions, some for prevention and some to treat headaches in progress. Eventually, I was put on verapamil [Calan, others], which I still take to this day; it seems to help. I was also put on gabapentin [Neurontin]. Those were preventive medications. In the meantime, I was given a prescription for Imitrex [sumatriptan] to treat individual events, but I switched to Relpax [eletriptan] because it doesn't give me heart palpitations and other side effects. It works great, but I know if I overuse it, it does have a rebound effect.

Having migraines does not preclude me from working as a pilot—it's the medications that matter. Now I only take medications that are approved for pilots. For example, I've been off gabapentin for seven or eight months now, because it's not on the approved list. I'm doing Botox every three months, which is approved for flight. I'm still taking the verapamil, and then the Relpax if I need it. I'm also taking supplements—a combination of turmeric, zinc, and magnesium—and I think I've seen good results with the turmeric particularly.

Being on Facebook groups is really helpful; people recommend things you'd never have thought of. There's no one perfect solution that works for everyone. I've been very lucky; I don't get auras or nausea. But it's hard. Every day is a question mark.

I've been called back to work, but I have a few months to decide whether I will go back. Most of my days are really good now, and my kids are more independent. I'm ready.

help people with both insomnia and chronic migraines.

Preventing recurrent headaches starts with simple pain relief treatments such as applying a heating pad daily to your neck and shoulders. You may want to consider physical therapy (ask your doctor for a referral), which often includes such techniques as massage, ultrasound, or gentle stretching to relieve muscle tightness that may precipitate further headaches (see "Physical therapy, massage, chiropractic, osteopathy," page 32). ♥

Cluster headaches

Cluster headaches deserve special mention because, although rare, they are among the most painful of all headaches. A typical cluster headache begins suddenly, often waking the person from sleep, most commonly between midnight and 2 a.m. The pain is intense, sharp, and penetrating, and it usually occurs behind one eye, which may be teary and bloodshot. The eyelid may droop, and the nostril on that side may first be stuffy and then runny. During a single attack, the symptoms will occur in either the left or right side, but never in both.

Unlike a person with a migraine headache—who tends to lie quietly in bed—someone having a cluster headache attack is likely to pace the floor. The pain is so excruciating that it's tempting to bang your head against a wall. After an hour or two, the pain and other symptoms usually recede, sometimes just as suddenly as they came on. But they tend to recur at the same time day after day.

About 10 times as many men as women have cluster headaches. About 90% of them have the episodic form: clusters of one or two headaches a day over a period of two to eight weeks, alternating with headache-free stretches. Usually, the remission time between cluster periods lasts six to 12 months, but it can be as short as a few weeks or as long as several years.

The other 10% of people with cluster headaches have attacks that continue for at least a year without any remission. These are known as chronic cluster headaches.

Managing cluster headaches

For immediate relief of cluster headaches, the most effective treatment is sumatriptan (Imitrex), which relieves about 75% of cluster headache attacks within 15 minutes when given by injection. The next most effective treatment is inhaling pure oxygen, administered in an emergency room or at home from a portable tank, which can be prescribed by a doctor. If there's no improvement after 15 minutes of inhaling, further oxygen therapy probably won't help. Injected DHE (see "Treating migraine pain," page 22) can quickly alleviate severe pain as well.

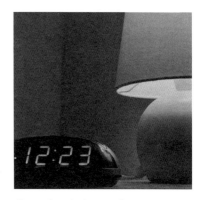

Cluster headaches tend to occur at the same time—usually between midnight and 2 a.m., making sleep during this time impossible.

Alcohol is a common trigger of cluster headaches, and avoiding it can help prevent them. The most effective preventive medications for cluster headaches are the calcium-channel blocker verapamil (Calan, others), the steroid prednisone, and the mood-stabilizing drug lithium. The average effective dose of verapamil for treating episodic cluster headaches—as much as 600 mg daily—is higher than that required to treat high blood pressure. The dose required for chronic cluster headaches is even higher—up to 1,200 mg a day. The higher the dose, the greater your risk of side effects, including low blood pressure, dizziness, and fainting.

High doses of steroids such as prednisone (60 to 80 mg per day) can also prevent further attacks when taken along with verapamil within 24 to 48 hours. Once you've interrupted the pattern, the steroids are stopped, but your doctor may continue to prescribe verapamil for a period of time as a preventive measure. The episodic form of cluster headache is more likely than the chronic form to respond to steroid therapy. ▼

Resources

Organizations

American Academy of Craniofacial Pain
11130 Sunrise Valley Drive, Suite 350
Reston, VA 20191
800-322-8651 (toll-free)
www.aacfp.org

This organization of health care professionals specializes in craniofacial pain and dysfunction. The website enables you to search for members near you.

American Academy of Orofacial Pain
174 S. New York Ave.
Oceanville, NJ 08231
609-504-1311
www.aaop.org

This organization of health care professionals specializes in orofacial pain and related disorders. You can search for members by state under the Patient Resources tab on the website.

American Headache Society
19 Mantua Road
Mt. Royal, NJ 08061
856-423-0043
americanheadachesociety.org

The American Headache Society is a professional society of health care providers that publishes information about the relief and prevention of headache, offers an online physician finder and a list of support groups, and sponsors public education campaigns.

American Society of Clinical Hypnosis
140 N. Bloomingdale Road
Bloomingdale, IL 60108
630-980-4740
www.asch.net

The website of this interdisciplinary organization of medical, dental, and mental health professionals allows you to search for providers by location and specialty; click on Member Referral Search under the Public tab.

National Certification Commission for Acupuncture and Oriental Medicine
76 S. Laura St., Suite 1290
Jacksonville, FL 32202
904-598-1005
www.nccaom.org

This nonprofit commission works to establish, assess, and promote standards of competence and safety in acupuncture and Oriental medicine. The website lets you search for providers in your area.

National Headache Foundation
820 N. Orleans, Suite 201
Chicago, IL 60610
312-274-2650
www.headaches.org

This nonprofit foundation provides information to people with headaches as well as to their families and health care providers. It publishes a bimonthly newsletter, a list of member physicians, and a variety of brochures and other educational materials for its members. The website also has useful information and links to related organizations.

National Institute of Neurological Disorders and Stroke (NINDS)
P.O. Box 5801
Bethesda, MD 20824
800-352-9424 (toll-free)
or 301-496-5751
www.ninds.nih.gov

This institute, part of the National Institutes of Health, provides a wealth of information on neurological disorders, including headache. Free informational booklets are published online and can be ordered by telephone. Search under "Disorders" on the NINDS website to find information about headache.

Society for Clinical & Experimental Hypnosis
P.O. Box 252
Southborough, MA 01772
508-598-5553
www.sceh.us

This international organization of health care professionals focuses on hypnosis research and clinical practice.

Glossary

aura: Neurological symptoms, such as flashing lights or a blind spot, that may precede a migraine headache.

biofeedback: A therapy that uses specialized devices to help individuals learn how to influence the function of organs or body systems that aren't usually thought to be under conscious control.

classic migraine: A migraine headache preceded by neurological symptoms that may include visual disturbances such as scintillations or a blind spot; now usually referred to as migraine with aura.

cluster headache: A severe headache on one side of the head, occurring as part of a series of similar attacks and lasting for an hour or two.

common migraine: A migraine headache not preceded by neurological symptoms; now usually referred to as migraine without aura.

computed tomography (CT): A diagnostic technique in which x-rays are taken from many different directions and a computer integrates the resulting data to produce cross-sectional images of body parts.

dihydroergotamine (DHE): a drug derived from certain types of fungus that's used in the treatment of migraines. DHE reduces migraine pain by constricting blood vessels.

ergots: Medications derived from a fungus that grows on rye and other grains; often used to treat headache.

ice-pick headache: A sudden, brief, severe stab of pain in the head.

magnetic resonance imaging (MRI): A diagnostic technique using powerful electromagnets, radiofrequency waves, and a computer to produce well-defined images of the body's internal structures.

migraine headache: A headache, usually occurring only on one side of the head, sometimes preceded by visual disturbances and often accompanied by nausea, vomiting, or sensitivity to light or noise.

neurotransmitter: A chemical that carries signals between brain cells.

nonsteroidal anti-inflammatory drug (NSAID): One of a class of drugs that reduce inflammation and pain.

paroxysmal hemicrania: A disorder resembling cluster headache, but with shorter and more frequent attacks.

ostia: Small openings that connect the sinuses to the nasal passages.

prodrome: Symptoms that precede a migraine headache by hours or days, including changes in mood, appetite, or activity level.

scintillation: The perception of flashing lights or lines that sometimes occurs during the aura of a migraine headache.

scotoma: A blank spot in the visual field that is sometimes evident during the aura of a migraine headache.

serotonin: A neurotransmitter that helps regulate sleep and appetite, mediate moods, and inhibit pain.

temporal arteritis: A condition involving inflammation of blood vessels; causes headache and sometimes leads to blindness.

tension headache: A headache, usually mild or moderate in intensity, not accompanied by other symptoms; pain is usually felt throughout the head, across the forehead, or in the back of the head.

thunderclap headache: A sudden, excruciating headache that may be the result of bleeding in the head.

tricyclics: A class of drugs that are thought to work by increasing the availability of serotonin and norepinephrine to nerve cell receptors. Often used in treating depression and other psychiatric problems.

trigger points: Very sensitive areas, usually in the back of the neck, that occur in some people with tension or migraine headaches; they are tender and, if touched, can prompt a headache.

triptans: A class of medications that work by constricting blood vessels in the head and perhaps by inhibiting inflammation.

vasoconstriction: narrowing of blood vessels resulting in restricted blood flow.

vasodilation: widening of blood vessels resulting in increased blood flow.

Notes